Interactive Cases in Emergency Medicine

This innovative book is based on real patients seen in the emergency department of a busy London teaching hospital. Developed from a project designed to offer an online alternative to in-person learning during the COVID-19 pandemic, the material will appeal to readers and educators seeking digital content to supplement traditional print-based learning resources. Seventy high-yield cases are illustrated with a variety of static images, including clinical photographs, radiographs and scans, blood films and ECG traces, coupled with integrated imaging videos to enhance understanding. Knowledge is tested via best of three questions, reflecting the format of qualifying examinations, while extensive answers provide further opportunities for learning and revision.

Reflecting both common and more complex clinical scenarios, the content will teach and challenge its readers, from the newly qualified resident doctor to more experienced clinicians and allied health personnel working in emergency and acute settings.

Interactive Cases Series

Series Editors: Dipak Mistry and Alice Yearwood

Interactive Cases in Emergency Medicine: Learning through Image Interpretation
Alice Yearwood & Dipak Mistry

https://www.routledge.com/Interactive-Cases-Series/book-series/CRCINTCASSER

Interactive Cases in Emergency Medicine
Learning through Image Interpretation

Edited by

Alice Yearwood MBBS iBSc(Hons)
Anaesthetic Resident
London, UK

Dipak Mistry MBBS BSc(Hons) DTM&H MRCS FRCEM
Consultant in Emergency Medicine
University College London Hospital
London, UK

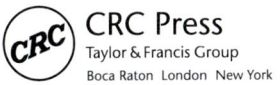

CRC Press
Taylor & Francis Group
Boca Raton London New York

CRC Press is an imprint of the
Taylor & Francis Group, an **informa** business

Designed cover image: Courtesy – Snehal Mistry; Book template source – Freepik (premium license)

First edition published 2026
by CRC Press
2385 NW Executive Center Drive, Suite 320, Boca Raton, FL 33431

and by CRC Press
4 Park Square, Milton Park, Abingdon, Oxon, OX14 4RN

CRC Press is an imprint of Taylor & Francis Group, LLC

ISBN: 9781032609942 (hbk)
ISBN: 9781032479842 (pbk)
ISBN: 9781003461456 (ebk)

DOI: 10.1201/9781003461456

Typeset in Univers LT Std
by Evolution Design & Digital Ltd.

To Marcos, for your unwavering support and reminding me what I am capable of.

Alice

To my wife, Snehal, for your endless support; to Shreya, Shailen and Shaan you are the future.

Dipak

Contents

Topic Key

GM	General Internal Medicine
ID	Infectious Diseases
T	Toxicology
NN	Neurology and Neurosurgery
TO	Trauma and Orthopaedics
EO	ENT, Ophthalmology and Maxillofacial Surgery
S	Surgery
P	Paediatrics
CC	Critical Care
OG	Obstetrics and Gynaecology
M	Medicolegal

Preface

The idea for *Interactive Cases in Emergency Medicine* was born from a seemingly small teaching initiative as the grip of a global pandemic threatened to derail the education programme for clinicians working in a central London emergency department (ED). It was clear that the traditional face-to-face teaching programme could not continue with the uncertainty of the rapidly changing clinical landscape and social distancing. We recognised the importance of being able to deliver quality educational sessions in a readily accessible format. Drawing on evidence-based educational techniques, a weekly mobile optimised case-based series was delivered throughout the pandemic and beyond, authored by clinicians working in the ED.

The following cases comprise of real patients who walked through the doors of our department. Each case is presented with three single best answer (SBA) questions, the style of which is encountered in many postgraduate examinations and is focused around one or more images from their clinical course. These images include not only static images but also video clips including CT, MRI and ultrasound. We have made these essential images accessible via a QR code and hope that you will review them in real time as if you were seeing the patient in the hospital. We hope that this hybrid learning helps to bring the cases to life and challenge both the novice and experienced clinician in Emergency Medicine. The answers are purposely short and originally served as a stimulus for discussion and we encourage you to read around the cases presented.

Finally, we would like to thank all of our original case authors for contributing and particinating in the original project bringing their unique perspectives and thought-provoking questions to our learning group. And most importantly, we thank our patients who are the focus of our clinical cases and central to our mission to improve care for everyone through education.

Alice Yearwood
Dipak Mistry

Contributors

Aashni Shah
Barbaros Sir
Charles Hensher
Christian Hesford
Cleodie Swire
Daniel Osikominu
Daniel Perelberg
Ed Deda
Emily Baker
Emma Johnson
Gil Bell
Greg Cameron
Hannah Ward
Jahnavi Panchal
Jai Adhupiya
James Sun
Jilan Patel
Joseph Jermy
Keshni Gudka
Maddy Tagg
Mahmood Soomro
Mahmuda Chadni
Marie Smith
Marwa Elamin
Mohammed Khoshkoo
Nabil George
Navroz Singh
Rachna Yamarthi
Raunak Poonawala
Samiha Ismail
Samit Patel
Samuel Williams
Saxon Hunt
Sindujen Sriharan
Sophie Eckersly
Thomas Perrin
Walid Ghandour
William Hull

CASE 1

A curiously high lactate

A 26-year-old woman presents to the emergency department (ED) in the early hours of the morning. She has been persistently vomiting for 3 days with two episodes of loose stools in the last 24 hours and states she 'can't keep anything down'. She tells you about a similar presentation to another hospital a month ago; she was told she had 'low blood sugar' and high lactate, which responded to intravenous (IV) fluid resuscitation, and she was discharged after a 14-hour stay in the ED. She denies being in contact with anyone who is unwell and has not eaten out or had takeaway meals. Her mother has type 2 diabetes mellitus and her sister has systemic lupus erythematosus.

Initial observations are recorded as HR 140, BP 128/65, SpO$_2$ 99% on room air RR 18, temperature 36.5°C (97.7°F), GCS 15/15. On examination, she looks unwell; her abdomen is distended and there is some vague tenderness in the epigastrium.

As part of the initial work-up, a venous blood gas (VBG) is taken.

Source	Venous		
pH	7.021∨	Oxyhaemoglobin %	17.4∨
Comment: Value below reference range		Comment: Value below reference range	
Carbon Dioxide Partial Pressure kPa	5.47	Saturated Oxygen %	17.8∨
Oxygen Partial Pressure kPa	3.06∨	Comment: Value below reference range	
Comment: Value below reference range		Carboxyhaemoglobin %	0.9
Potassium mmol/L	4.2	Methaemoglobin %	1.2
Sodium mmol/L	139	Bilirubin micromol/l	25∧
Ionised Calcium mmol/L	1.10∨	Comment: Value above reference range	
Comment: Value below reference range		Standard Base Excess mmol/L	−20.3∨
Chloride mmol/L	104	Comment: Value below reference range	
Glucose mmol/L	2.0∨	Standard Bicarbonate mmol/L	9.3∨
Comment: Value below reference range		Comment: Value below reference range	
Lactate mmol/L	18∧	Haematocrit %	40.4
Comment: Value above reference range		Oxygen Tension at 50% Saturation kPa	5.55
Urea mmol/L	5.9	Oxygen Content mmol/L	1.5
Creatinine micromol/l	63.8		
Total Haemoglobin g/l	132		

DOI: 10.1201/9781003461456-1

1. Which of the following could best explain the observed result?
   a. Primary adrenal insufficiency
   b. Pancreatitis
   c. Starvation ketoacidosis
   d. Metformin overdose
   e. Renal tubular acidosis

The patient is resuscitated with IV balanced crystalloid fluid and the lactate reduces to 13.9 after 4 L.

Laboratory blood tests are reviewed showing:

> Hb 129, WCC 15.34, plt 576, Cr 56, ALT 302, ALP 93, bilirubin 26, albumin 29, amylase 27, CRP 11, INR 2.27

The patient is admitted to the intensive care unit (ICU).

An abdominal USS is performed, which is reported as follows:

> 'Reversal of flow within the portal vein and no visible colour Doppler flow within the hepatic veins. Intrahepatic tortuosities, which may be consistent with venous collaterals. Large-volume ascites.'

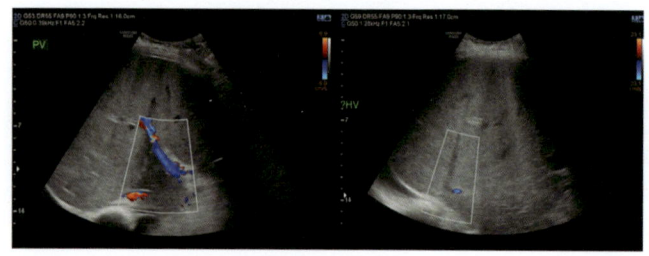

2. Which of the following conditions best accounts for this appearance on ultrasound?
   a. Arnold–Chiari syndrome
   b. Budd–Chiari syndrome
   c. Hepato-renal syndrome
   d. Hepatic artery aneurysm
   e. Inferior vena cava thrombus

3. Which of the following conditions is the most common cause of the underlying hepatic diagnosis (not necessarily for this patient)?

   a. Hepatocellular carcinoma

   b. Polycythaemia vera

   c. Pregnancy

   d. Use of oral contraceptives

   e. Factor V Leiden mutation

☑ 1d Metformin overdose

All of the options presented could cause a metabolic acidosis. When determining a cause of metabolic acidosis, it is useful to divide the causes into: (1) increased acid production, for example, lactic acidosis, diabetic/starvation/alcoholic ketoacidosis, ethanol/methanol/ethylene glycol poisoning; (2) loss of bicarbonate ions, for example, GI losses in diarrhoea and vomiting; or (3) failure of tubular bicarbonate reabsorption, for example, renal tubular acidosis. Note that alongside the raised anion gap metabolic acidosis with extremely high lactate seen here is hypoglycaemia. Of the provided options, metformin overdose could present this result. Metformin blocks the first step of gluconeogenesis by inhibiting pyruvate carboxylase, which causes an accumulation of lactic acid. Alternatively severe paracetamol overdose, ethanol poisoning, ethylene glycol poisoning could also explain the observed result. In non-diabetic individuals, such a profound hypoglycaemia would be unusual in starvation ketoacidosis. Pancreatitis with significant vomiting could cause a normal anion gap metabolic acidosis with hypoglycaemia.

☑ 2b Budd–Chiari syndrome

The correct answer is Budd–Chiari syndrome, which is caused by either partial or complete occlusion of the hepatic veins. Classically, it presents with the clinical triad of abdominal pain, hepatomegaly and ascites. The liver is unique in that it receives a dual inflow from the hepatic portal vein (70%) and hepatic artery (30%). When the hepatic veins thrombose, the liver engorges with blood, causing hepatomegaly and ascites. The obstruction results in reversal of flow in the hepatic portal vein (hepatofugal – literally 'fleeing' the liver), which can be picked up on Doppler or colour flow USS. Other sonographic features include absent flow in the hepatic veins due to thrombus, low flow or bidirectional flow in the IVC and hepatic venous collaterals. The diagnosis may be further confirmed with a portal venous phase contrast CT of the abdomen and pelvis, which this patient went on to have whilst in ICU.

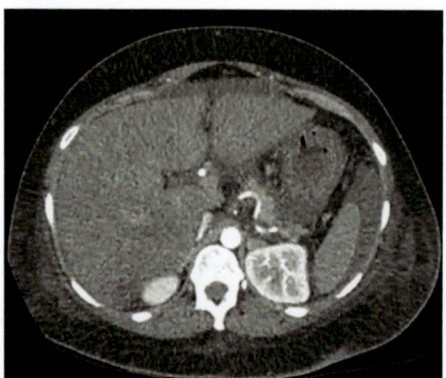

☑ 3b Polycythaemia vera

Budd–Chiari syndrome is associated with prothrombotic states and so all the answers here are potential underlying causes, but almost 10% of cases are caused by polycythaemia vera. Around 75% of cases result from thrombosis within the hepatic veins, whereas 25% arise from external compression that results in obstruction. All of the above answers produce a physiological hypercoagulable state and should be considered when investigating for a cause, though it is thought that approximately one third of cases with hepatic venous thrombosis are idiopathic. Management tends to be based on treating any underlying cause and a stepwise approach with medical management (anticoagulation, thrombolytics, diuretics), endovascular treatment to restore vessel patency (angioplasty, stenting and local thrombolysis), on to transjugular intrahepatic portosystemic shunt (TIPS) or liver transplantation if decompensated cirrhosis is present. Untreated, the syndrome has a mortality of 80%.

KEY LEARNING POINTS

- When considering the causes of a metabolic acidosis, calculating an anion gap and using a medical sieve can be helpful in determining the underlying cause.
- The liver has a unique dual incoming blood supply arranged in a functional unit known as a portal triad consisting of the majority from the hepatic portal vein and the remainder from the hepatic artery.
- Alterations in hepatic blood flow due to Virchow's triad (venous stasis, vascular injury or hypercoagulability) may result in thrombosis.

CASE 2

A cycling wrist injury

A 59-year-old man presents 5 hours after a cycling accident where he fell onto his left side after his bicycle wheel clipped the kerb. He complains of significant bruising, swelling and pain in his left hand and wrist, which is worsening despite using ice packs and simple analgesia.

Radiographs are requested.

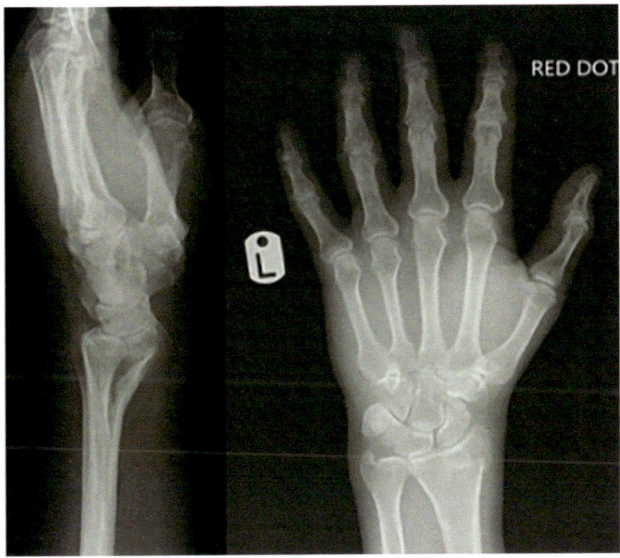

RED DOT

1. Which of the following is the most common injury mechanism leading to the above fracture pattern?

    a. Fall onto a flexed wrist

    b. Forced dorsiflexion and abduction of the hand

    c. Fall onto an outstretched hand with bent elbow

    d. Fall onto an outstretched hand

    e. Fall onto an abducted thumb

DOI: 10.1201/9781003461456-2

This fracture pattern can impair the median nerve as it runs through the carpal tunnel in the wrist.

2. Which of the following best describes how to assess the neurological status of this nerve?

   a. Sensation to the volar thumb, index, middle and lateral half of ring finger and associated palm area; thumb opposition and flexion of index and middle fingers

   b. Sensation to the volar aspect of the little finger and half of ring finger and associated palm area; finger adduction

   c. Sensation to the volar thumb, index, middle and half of ring finger and associated palm area; finger abduction and adduction

   d. Sensation to the volar aspect of the little finger and half of ring finger and associated palm area; thumb opposition and flexion of index and middle fingers

   e. Sensation to the dorsal aspect of lateral hand and thumb including the anatomical snuffbox; thumb adduction

Following reduction under haematoma block, a CT is performed with 3D reconstructions.

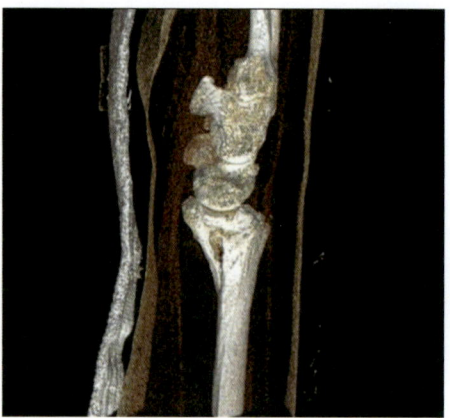

The patient reports numbness in the thumb and index finger and reduced movement but thinks this could be due to the local anaesthetic. The fingers appear pink and warm to palpation.

3. Which of the following is the best option in terms of the next step in management?

    a. Refer to the orthopaedic resident for second attempt at reduction

    b. Discharge from emergency department (ED) with referral to fracture clinic; advise sensation will return as local anaesthetic wears off

    c. Release the cast down to skin longitudinally, elevate with a Bradford sling and refer to the orthopaedic registrar on-call

    d. Elevate the hand on two blankets and perform hourly motor and sensory checks until the anaesthetic wears off

    e. Refer to the physiotherapy and occupational therapy team for functional assessment prior to discharge

☑ 1d Fall onto an outstretched hand

The radiograph shows an impacted, intra-articular fracture of the left distal radius with volar displacement best seen on the lateral view (note the position of the lunate). This fracture pattern, commonly referred to as a 'volar Barton's fracture', is often caused by a fall onto an outstretched hand (FOOSH) in pronation. FOOSH with an extended elbow commonly leads to a Colle's fracture (distal radius fracture with dorsal angulation) or scaphoid fracture, whereas FOOSH with a flexed elbow may lead to a Galeazzi fracture-dislocation (distal radial fracture with dislocation of the distal radioulnar joint and an intact ulna). Forced dorsiflexion and abduction of the hand may lead to intra-articular fracture of the radial styloid, sometimes referred to as a Hutchinson or chauffeur fracture. Fall onto an abducted thumb can result in a Bennett fracture (oblique two-piece fracture of the base of thumb metacarpal with intra-articular extension) or a Rolando fracture (comminuted fracture at the base of the thumb metacarpal).

☑ 2a Sensation to the volar thumb, index, middle and lateral half of ring finger and associated palm area; thumb opposition and flexion of index and middle fingers

A volar Barton's fracture can lead to damage to the median nerve at the level of the wrist. Therefore, the correct options are to assess for sensory change over the volar aspect of the lateral three and a half fingers and associated palm area and assess motor function thumb opposition and flexion of index and middle fingers. The ulnar nerve distribution is sensation to the volar aspect of the little finger and medial half of the ring finger and associated palm and dorsum of hand. Motor function can be tested by thumb and finger adduction. The radial nerve distribution provides sensation to dorsal aspect of thumb, index, middle and lateral half of ring finger and associated dorsum of hand. Motor function can be tested by finger extension (note that the radial nerve supplies muscles of the arm and forearm). A really quick way to assess motor function of the nerves to the hand is to ask the patient to perform 'rock, paper, scissors, OK' signs with their hand – it's effective in both children and adults and has been well validated in literature.

☑ 3c Release the cast down to skin longitudinally, elevate with a Bradford sling and refer to the orthopaedic registrar on-call

Any fractures with suggestions of neurovascular compromise should be reviewed urgently in the ED by the on-call orthopaedic registrar. The main concern with this injury pattern is compression of the median nerve, which is a potential cause of this patient's ongoing sensory disturbance. The CT 3D reconstruction shows a large bony fragment displaced in a volar direction (0m18s). This puts pressure on the median nerve causing a neuropraxia. Sometimes extensive haematoma will also cause compression of the median nerve. Always check to see if the cast is tight and release the bandage including velband (i.e. down to skin) to see if symptoms improve. Note the volar backslab as seen in the CT reconstructions, not the more commonly applied dorsal cast. Another attempt at reduction might improve the position along with elevation in a Bradford sling. However, these patients should be referred early to the orthopaedic registrar or consultant as they may need emergent open reduction and internal fixation along with a carpal tunnel decompression. In this case, the patient went to theatre immediately for an open reduction and internal fixation (ORIF) and carpal tunnel release and there was a large haematoma compressing the median nerve in the carpal tunnel. Post-operatively, he regained full median nerve function and did very well.

KEY LEARNING POINTS

- A careful history with attention to the mechanism of injury will help to predict fracture patterns and associated injuries.
- Neurovascular assessment should be documented down to the individual nerve and artery, especially prior to any interventions.
- 'Rock, paper, scissors, OK!' is an effective and swift method of testing motor function of the median, radial and ulnar nerve in both adults and children.
- In the case of neurovascular compromise, prompt referral to a senior surgeon is key.

CASE 3

A deformed arm after falling on the train

A 10-year-old boy presents to the emergency department (ED) with his mother. They are visiting from the USA and arrived only yesterday. This afternoon they were travelling on the London Underground when the train moved forwards to depart from a station and the patient fell over, landing with full force onto his left forearm. He did not sustain a head injury and remembers the event clearly. There was an immediate deformity to his forearm. Past medical history includes two previous fractures to the same forearm; he was investigated by paediatricians in the USA and had tests that were reported as normal. He is not on any regular medicines and is not allergic to anything.

You assess him in triage with one of the paediatric nurses who has already given ibuprofen 300 mg and paracetamol 500 mg.

Initial observations are recorded as HR 78, BP 100/56, SpO_2 98% on room air, RR 28, temperature 37.1°C (98.78°F). The patient reports his pain score as 11 out of 10.

Screening primary survey is as follows:

Airway + c-spine: no cervical spine pain noted

Breathing: chest has good air entry bilaterally, there is no pain to the chest wall

Circulation: heart sounds normal, no abdominal pain

Disability: GCS 15/15, no signs of head injury

Exposure: there is an obvious deformity to the left forearm

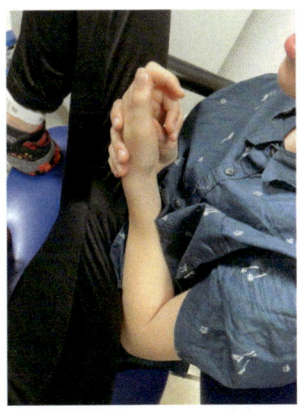

DOI: 10.1201/9781003461456-3

You want to perform a basic distal neurovascular examination but the patient is very distressed, as is his mother.

1. Which of the following analgesia options is the next best choice for this patient?

    a. Diamorphine intranasal 4 mg

    b. Entonox inhaled PRN

    c. Penthrox inhaled PRN

    d. Heliox inhaled PRN

    e. Codeine phosphate 60 mg PO

You discuss the case with the attending ED consultant who tells you to perform a screening motor exam using the 'rock, paper, scissors, OK!' method. They also remind you to double check the anterior interosseous nerve (AIN) as this can be injured in forearm fractures.

Radiographs are performed.

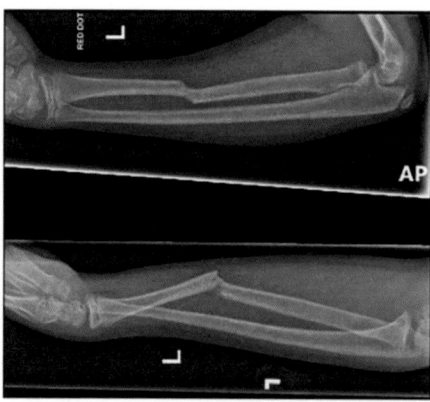 

2. Which muscle or group does the AIN innervate and what hand movement would the patient NOT be able to do if damaged by the injury in the radiograph above?

    a. Finger flexors (Rock sign)

    b. Finger extensors (Paper sign)

    c. Finger abductors (Scissors sign)

    d. Flexor policis longus and flexor digitorum profundus (OK sign)

    e. Biceps contraction (Guns out sign)

Based on your clinical examination, which confirms this is an isolated injury, you place a cannula on the opposite side and order blood tests.

The orthopaedic team assess the patient and take him to theatre. There, a closed reduction is attempted but the fracture is very unstable. Based on this, the following operation is performed.

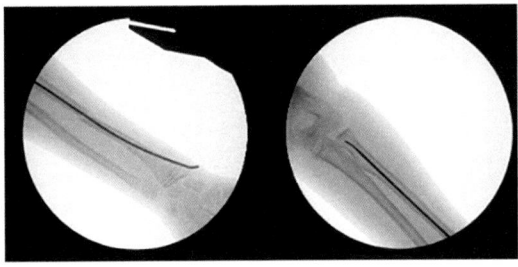 

3. What is the name of the device inserted to ensure a stable reduction?

   a. Kirschner wire fixation

   b. Titanium Elastic Nailing System (TENS)

   c. Ilizarov frame

   d. Halo system

   e. Intramedullary locking nail

☑ 1a Diamorphine intranasal 4 mg

The best analgesic option is intranasal diamorphine for this patient. When assessing any patient with an injury, good analgesia should be given in proportion to the injury sustained and should follow the WHO pain ladder wherever possible. In this patient, we have a significant injury and a very high pain score. Baseline paracetamol and ibuprofen have already been administered and therefore a strong opioid is required to ensure he is made more comfortable. Diamorphine intranasally does not require the presence of a cannula and is an attractive option for rapid-onset analgesia. The dose is 0.1 mg/kg (rounded up to 4 mg in this instance), which is administered via an atomiser to the nostril whilst the child sniffs. Onset of action can be as fast as IV administration and the analgesic effects can last up to an hour in some cases. Respiratory depression is very rarely seen, but children require monitoring following administration and particular care should be taken in head injuries. Considering the incorrect options, codeine is a weak opioid which is not licensed in the under 12s. Entonox® (50/50 mix of oxygen/nitrus oxide) is only very short lived and can induce euphoria. It can be useful for very short procedures such as dressing changes. Penthrox® is the brand name for methoxyflurane which is delivered by a patient-administered inhalational device. It tends to be easier to use than Entonox but is not currently licensed for use in those under 18 years. The dose lasts for approximately 30 minutes, starting after about 6–8 breaths and continues for several minutes after stopping inhalation. Heliox is not an analgesic. It is a mixture of helium and oxygen and is used mostly in head and neck cancer patients who have difficulty breathing due to its lower resistance passing through the respiratory tract, requiring less effort by the patient.

☑ 2d Flexor policis longus and flexor digitorum profundus (OK sign)

Injury to the AIN can be from both supracondylar fractures and forearm diaphysis fractures, and results in the loss of the ability in performing the 'OK' hand sign. As well as the two muscles above, the anterior interosseous nerve also innervates the pronator quadratus. When assessing neurology, it is more helpful to document individual nerve function. In paediatrics, the game 'rock, paper, scissors' provides a really good screening test with the addition of the 'OK' sign. The finger flexors are innervated by the median nerve and this is tested by making a fist. Wrist extension and extension at the metacarpophalangeal joints are controlled by the radial nerve, which is tested by the paper movement. Finger adduction and abduction is controlled by the ulnar nerve, and this is tested by the scissor movement. Finally, as above, the AIN is tested by the 'OK' sign. Don't forget to document the sensory component as well as both the radial and ulnar artery pulses.

☑ 3b Titanium Elastic Nailing System (TENS)

Unlike adults, children may not tolerate attempts at closed reduction in the ED and this needs to be performed under a general anaesthetic in theatre with screening radiographs. As a general principle for reducing fractures, traction in the long axis of the bone will reduce most fractures and dislocations. If the fracture is stable, it can be immobilised in the reduced position to allow for appropriate union. In this case, the fracture was unstable despite reduction, so fixation was required to hold the bones in the appropriate position to heal. When thinking about options for fixation of a fracture, these can be divided into external and internal fixation. External fixation is most commonly used in the stabilisation of open fractures, severely comminuted and unstable fractures, fractures associated with infection or non-union, and severe soft tissue injuries. Devices such as the Ilizarov frame (lower leg) and Halo system (cervical spine) are used for external fixation. Internal fixation options can be further classified by extramedullary devices such as wires, plates and screws, versus intramedullary nailing. Kirschner wires ('K-wires') are deformable metal wires used for fixation of fractures in epi-/metaphyseal areas, fractures of small bones, small fracture fragments and fragment reposition in multi-fragmentary fractures, in addition to stable fixation. They are generally removed once adequate healing has occurred. In this patient a specialised intramedullary nailing system – TENS – was deployed to achieve a very good result. The TENS nail is placed to avoid the growth plates and removed after 4–6 months after full healing has been achieved. A traditional intramedullary locking nail permits placement of locking screws through bone and nail, to improve fixation proximally and distally. In a child this is contraindicated as it would not allow ongoing growth to the limb.

KEY LEARNING POINTS

- Intranasal diamorphine is a rapidly acting, extremely effective strong opioid analgesia for paediatric patients who are in severe pain.
- Following reduction, if the fracture remains unstable it requires fixation to ensure good union and reduce risk of functional impairment.
- There are many options for both external and internal fixation depending on injury location and additional injury characteristics; this is often determined following discussion in specific trauma meetings with multiple orthopaedic senior staff.
- The Titanium Elastic Nailing System (TENS) is an intramedullary nail system used in children that allows ongoing growth to the limb.

CASE 4

A gardener's eye

A 26-year-old man with no past medical or medication history presents to the emergency department with anisocoria. He denies sustaining any trauma and has no eye pain, vomiting, headache, dizziness, confusion or loss of consciousness. He denies recreational drug use and is a non-smoker. His observations are all within normal limits and he appears well.

His pupils are as pictured. The left pupil demonstrates a normal light reflex, but the right has very little movement.

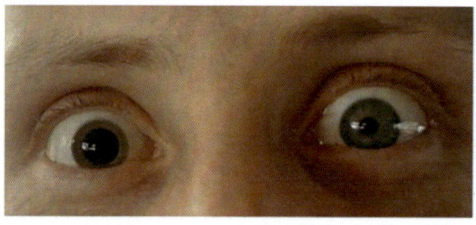 

1.   Which of the following would be unlikely to be associated with anisocoria?
     a.   Pituitary tumour
     b.   Direct eye trauma
     c.   Major head trauma
     d.   Intracranial mass lesion
     e.   Holmes–Adie pupil

On further questioning he states he was gardening and cutting *Brugmansia suaveolens*, commonly known as Angel's trumpet.

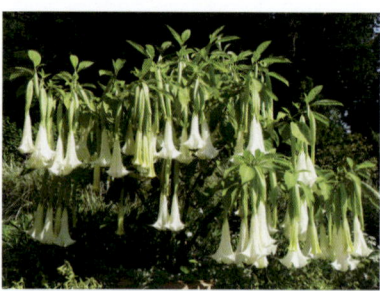 

DOI: 10.1201/9781003461456-4

2. What compound found in this plant could account for this presentation?

    a. Pilocarpine

    b. Vinca alkaloids (vincristine, vinblastine)

    c. Physostigmine

    d. Tropane alkaloids (scopolamine, atropine)

    e. Bolesatine

You have performed a comprehensive eye exam that does not show any other abnormality.

3. How will you proceed?

    a. Discharge and advise to return if not improving within 24 hours

    b. Instil pilocarpine drops immediately and refer to ophthalmology

    c. Arrange a CT of the head with contrast

    d. Refer to acute internal medicine for admission and sit 60-degrees head-up

    e. Give chloramphenicol eye drops QDS for 5–7 days

☑ 1a Pituitary tumour

Pituitary tumours typically cause pressure on the optic nerve causing bitemporal hemi-anopia and so are not usually associated with anisocoria. In contrast, direct eye trauma, conditions that raise ICP, such as intracranial bleeds or mass lesions and a Holmes–Adie pupil can all cause anisocoria. Other causes of unilateral dilated pupil include oculomo-tor nerve lesions/palsy, eye pathologies, Miller–Fisher syndrome (considered a variant of Guillain–Barré syndrome), diabetes, multiple sclerosis, multiple system atrophy and drugs. Considering Holmes–Adie pupil in a bit more detail, the pupil is typically dilated and sluggish in its response to direct light. The exact cause of a Holmes–Adie pupil is unknown but may be related to inflammation or damage to the ciliary ganglion or post-ganglionic nerve fibres. It typically affects females more than males and is most common between the ages of 25 and 45. In some individuals, there are also absent or sluggish deep tendon reflexes as well and this is referred to as Holmes–Adie syndrome.

☑ 2d Tropane alkaloids (scopolamine, atropine)

Brugmansia suaveolens (Angel's trumpet) is rich in scopolamine, hyoscyamine and atro-pine, all of which have anti-cholinergic effects. Localised antagonism of the parasym-pathetic muscarinic acetylcholine receptors leads to paralysis of the smooth muscle in the pupillary sphincter and ciliary muscles and therefore mydriasis (pupillary dilatation). Acetylcholine receptor antagonists, often termed anti-cholinergic or anti-muscarinic drugs, reduce the action of the parasympathetic nervous system, whose actions can be remembered by the mnemonic SLUDGE (**S**alivation, **L**acrimation, **U**rination, **D**efecation, **G**I upset, **E**mesis). These drugs can also have central effects typically leading to hyper-active delirium with agitation, confusion, restlessness and hallucinations. Looking at the other options, pilocarpine is an agonist at muscarinic acetylcholine receptors leading to miosis and is used in primary angle closure glaucoma as the opening of the trabec-ular meshwork allows aqueous humour to drain from the anterior compartment. Vinca alkaloids are used in chemotherapy and are found in *Catharanthus roseus* (periwinkle plant). Bolesatine is found in the Satan's bolete mushroom and causes severe GI effects if eaten. Physostigmine is an acetyl-cholinesterase inhibitor used to treat systemic alka-loid poisoning.

☑ 3a Discharge and advise to return if not improving within 24 hours

The anti-cholinergic effects of *Brugmansia suaveolens* are reported to last about 24–48 hours; therefore, this patient should be advised to return if anisocoria persists beyond this. *Brugmansia suaveolens*-induced mydriasis will in most cases self-resolve and rou-tine follow-up is not needed. However, lower your threshold for referral if the patient is older or has glaucoma, as intraocular pressure may need to be monitored. Instillation of pilocarpine will not reverse a pharmacologically dilated pupil as in this case. Antibiotic eye drops such as chloramphenicol are not indicated even as prophylaxis. Anisocoria is thought to affect up to 20% of the population and as aforementioned the causes can range from benign conditions to those that are much more serious. The key to the diagnosis, as always, is a detailed history, examination and appropriate investigations as indicated. History should include onset and chronicity, presence of headache, ptosis, diplopia, numbness, weakness ataxia, as well as ophthalmic history, presence of co-morbidities, contact with topical medications or other exposures. Physical examination includes presence of ptosis, ophthalmoplegias and pupillary response to light and accommodation. If there are any inconsistencies with assessment, it is suggested to seek expert ophthalmological opinion.

KEY LEARNING POINTS

- A careful eye history should include occupation and recreational hobbies as this may yield clues to inadvertent topical exposure or injury.
- Think carefully in a stepwise manner when thinking about pupillary or visual abnormalities, i.e. structural globe abnormalities, retina, receptors and conductive system leading to central nervous system including ganglia.
- In cases where topical poisoning is suspected, expert help from both a toxicologist and ophthalmologist can clarify management steps, including prognosis, and provide a robust safety net.

CASE 5

A painful foot

A 60-year-old man presents with left foot and ankle pain. He attended the emergency department (ED) 2 weeks earlier with a left ankle inversion injury. Radiographs performed at that time were normal and he was discharged without routine follow-up. Since then, his pain has worsened and so he returned to the ED. On direct questioning, he denies sensory changes, paraesthesia or weakness to the foot or ankle. He has no significant past medical history but does report a 40-pack year smoking history.

On examination, the left foot is tender over the lateral malleolus, there is no obvious swelling or bruising, the foot is pink and capillary refill time is less than 2 seconds. Sensation is intact. The dorsalis pedis and posterior tibial pulses are not palpable.

1. Which artery directly supplies the dorsalis pedis artery?
   a. Anterior tibial artery
   b. Peroneal artery
   c. Popliteal artery
   d. Posterior tibial artery
   e. Anterior lateral malleolar artery

You attempt to locate the dorsalis pedis and posterior tibial pulses with a handheld Doppler and find a monophasic flow.

A CT angiogram of the lower limbs is therefore performed.

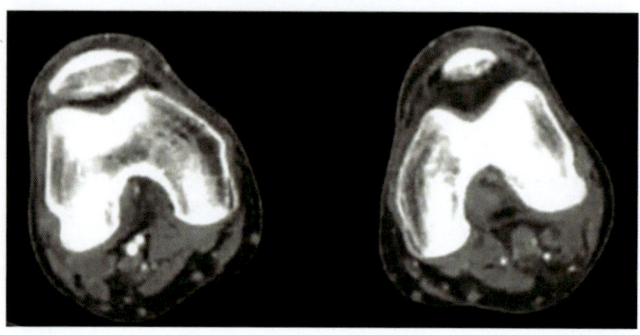

DOI: 10.1201/9781003461456-5

2. What does the CT angiogram show?

    a. Fracture of the distal left fibula

    b. Left popliteal artery aneurysm

    c. Occlusion of the left anterior tibial artery

    d. Occlusion of the left tibioperoneal trunk

    e. Occlusion of the left femoral artery

3. Based on the findings on the CT angiogram, what is the most appropriate management within the ED?

    a. Discharge with analgesia, aircast boot and GP follow-up

    b. Refer to the orthopaedic registrar on-call to consider fasciotomy

    c. Anticoagulate with unfractionated heparin and arrange urgent referral to vascular surgeons

    d. Discharge with analgesia, request an outpatient ultrasound duplex scan and routine referral to outpatient vascular clinic

    e. Discharge with dual antiplatelet therapy (for example, aspirin and clopidogrel), statin and tramadol, and routine referral to outpatient vascular clinic

☑ 1a Anterior tibial artery

The anterior tibial artery is the direct supply to the dorsalis pedis artery. The main arterial supply to the lower limb is the femoral artery as a continuation of the external iliac artery once it crosses under the inguinal ligament into the femoral triangle. This passes down the anterior aspect of the thigh, through a tunnel known as the adductor canal, then passes posteriorly through the adductor hiatus (Hunter's canal) entering the popliteal fossa where it becomes the popliteal artery. The popliteal artery ends by dividing into the anterior tibial artery and the tibioperoneal trunk. In turn, the tibioperoneal trunk bifurcates into the posterior tibial and peroneal arteries. The peroneal artery supplies the lateral compartment of the lower leg via perforating branches. The posterior tibial artery passes along the surface of deep posterior leg muscles and enters the sole of the foot via the tarsal tunnel, accompanying the tibial nerve. The anterior tibial artery passes anteriorly through a gap in the interosseous membrane running down the length of the lower leg and into the foot where it becomes the dorsalis pedis artery.

☑ 2d Occlusion of the left tibioperoneal trunk

The CT angiogram of the lower limbs shows occlusion of the left tibioperoneal trunk just below the end point of the popliteal artery. This can be seen by loss of contrast visualised in the left side around the level of the proximal tibia. You can also appreciate some collateral vessels present within the lower left leg (seen as highly attenuating vessels due to the contrast), suggesting a degree of chronic ischaemia. The imaged arteries in the right lower leg were normal, although the patient was found to have a thrombus in the right internal iliac artery (not seen in this video). Classically, signs and symptoms of acute limb ischaemia can be described using the 6 Ps: **P**ain, **P**ulselessness, **P**allor, **P**araesthesia, **P**erishingly cold, **P**aralysis. The first three symptoms tend to be the most common, but as you can see not all patients will present in a classical sense and with our patient this may be due to the likely acute-on-chronic presentation. The Rutherford classification categorises acute limb ischaemia into categories and prognoses based on clinical features or sensory loss, motor deficit, arterial and venous Dopplers.

☑ 3c Anticoagulate with unfractionated heparin and arrange urgent referral to vascular surgeons

This patient has acute limb ischaemia with threatened tissue viability and should be urgently reviewed by a vascular surgeon. In this instance, the limb is still viable (no significant tissue loss, nerve damage or significant sensory loss) and should undergo revascularisation either endovascularly or surgically. Immediate management in the ED includes analgesia, anticoagulation with unfractionated heparin, with oxygen and IV fluids if indicated. There is no specific recommended analgesia for ischaemia but high analgesic requirements including IV opioids are likely to be required as part of a multi-modal approach. NSAIDs should be avoided in vasculopaths due to risk of myocardial events. Heparin is usually given even if likely to be undergoing surgery or angiography to prevent propagation of thrombosis; options include both low molecular weight heparin and unfractionated heparin. Remember to discuss this with the vascular surgeon during referral. Delays in referral risk jeopardising the limb in these patients and familiarity with local vascular centre policies is advisable; be aware that prehospital and transport services may not be able to transport patients on heparin infusion compared to paramedics.

KEY LEARNING POINTS

- When examining joints, do not forget to perform a screening neurovascular examination comparing one side to another.
- A working knowledge of anatomy is essential to interpret scans such as CT angiograms and will allow rapid and early identification of gross pathology.
- Patients with vascular emergencies may be present in an atypical manner but persistent pain is a prominent feature.
- Remember to review your local referral pathways for vascular patients, especially if working in remote areas or where services may be centralised (hub and spoke centres).

A painful rash

An 18-year-old man presents to the emergency department (ED) in a central London hospital with a 5-day history of painful skin lesions, predominantly affecting his hands, feet and mouth. He initially felt generally unwell with fevers and is now struggling to eat and drink due to mucosal pain. He reported an episode of a 'sore throat' around 2 weeks prior to the lesions appearing, which was treated with a course of co-amoxiclav from a different hospital; the rash started on day 6 of the 7-day course. He is otherwise fit and well with no past medical history. He has no known allergies.

Initial observations are recorded as HR 111, BP 125/75, RR 24, SpO$_2$ 100% on room air, temperature 39.5°C (103.1°F).

You observe multiple lesions across the hands and feet and on the oral mucosa.

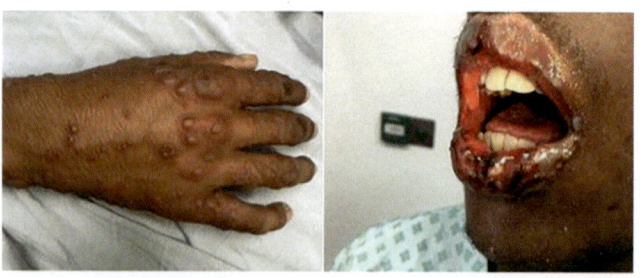 

1. Which set of investigations would you initially order in the ED?
   a. Draw bloods (FBC/U&E/CRP/HIV), blood cultures, chest radiograph, urine dip and culture
   b. Draw bloods (FBC/U&E/CRP/HIV) only
   c. Draw bloods (FBC/U&E/CRP), chest radiograph, urine dip, respiratory viral throat swab
   d. Draw bloods (FBC/U&E/CRP/HIV), blood cultures, bacterial MC&S and NAAT throat swab
   e. Draw bloods (FBC/U&E), urine dip, bacterial MC&S and NAAT throat swab

You refer to the acute internal medicine team for admission for further investigation.

They ask you to calculate the Score of TEN (SCORTEN) score.

DOI: 10.1201/9781003461456-6

2. Which of the following is one of the variables required to calculate this?
   a. Sex
   b. Blood pressure
   c. Creatinine
   d. Lactate
   e. Bicarbonate

The dermatology team are consulted, who suggest several other tests.

3. Which of the following further investigations would NOT help to differentiate the diagnosis?
   a. Viral screen (including HSV, VZV, EBV, CMV, viral hepatitis)
   b. Mycoplasma serology
   c. Bacterial throat swab
   d. Autoimmune screen (including ANA, ANCA, ENA)
   e. Skin biopsy

☑ 1a Draw bloods (FBC/U&E/CRP/HIV), blood cultures, chest radiograph, urine dip and culture

At their initial presentation, any patient presenting with potential signs of sepsis (fever, tachycardia, tachypnoea) should have a full work-up, including blood work for inflammatory markers, renal function and septic screen with blood cultures, chest radiograph and urine dip as a minimum. In areas where local HIV prevalence is ≥2/1000, routine HIV testing should be considered. There are certainly further investigations that can then be considered, such as throat swabs, swabs of lesions and additional blood tests as indicated. Looking at the rash present in the photo above, some of the lesions appear bullous, and others appear almost target-like. The differentials for this rash are wide, but the involvement of mucosal membranes should warn you to consider Stevens–Johnson syndrome (SJS)/Toxic Epidermal Necrolysis (TEN) or erythema multiforme (EM). SJS/TEN are now thought to be variants of the same condition, which is distinct from erythema multiforme. SJS/TEN is a rare condition but potentially fatal and is a dermatological emergency. It can be the result of medication use and it develops unpredictably in any age group and ethnicity in anyone on any medication. It is 100 times more common in association with HIV infection. The fever and systemic upset in this case could be due to an inflammatory rather than infective process in this instance, but it would be prudent to cover with antibiotics once samples for culture have been taken initially until infection is excluded.

☑ 2e Bicarbonate

The SCORTEN score is an illness severity score developed to predict mortality in SJS and TEN cases. One point is scored for each of the seven criteria present at the time of admission. These criteria are: age >40 years, presence of malignancy, heart rate >120 bpm, initial percentage of epidermal detachment >10% BSA, urea >10 mmol/L, glucose >14 mmol/L and bicarbonate <20 mmol/L. Base excess is not involved in SCORTEN calculation. Mortality significantly increases from 3.2% if 0–1, to 12.1% if 2, up to >90% if 5 or more. A more recent prediction model called the ABCD-10 was proposed in 2019: Age >50 (1 point), Bicarbonate <20 (1 point), Cancer (2 points), Dialysis prior to admission (3 points), Epidermal detachment >10% BSA. However, further validation of this scoring system is still required.

☑ 3c Bacterial throat swab

Expert opinion is needed to determine the exact diagnosis in this instance, but the main differentials are erythema multiforme major or SJS/TEN spectrum. The most common precipitant for SJS/TEN is a drug reaction. It usually occurs within a week of the offending antibiotic, but within 2 months of anticonvulsants. However, infections are associated with at least 90% of cases of EM. The single most common trigger for

EM is herpes simplex infection (usually herpes labialis); mycoplasma is the next most common. Some drugs can also precipitate EM, including antibiotics, anticonvulsants, NSAIDs and some immunisations. A full viral screen and mycoplasma serology should be sent to assess for presence of these. An autoimmune screen may also be useful in cases of no obvious infective precipitant. Additionally, a skin biopsy may be required to guide diagnosis. Management of EM is generally supportive, ensuring adequate analgesia for skin lesions and oral pain, antihistamines or steroids for pruritus and involving ophthalmology in case of eye symptoms.

This patient was diagnosed with erythema multiforme, for which he had previously seen dermatology a few months previously. It was suspected to be triggered by a mycoplasma infection. He was admitted due to severity of oral lesions and inability to maintain hydration. Herpes simplex virus is a more common cause of recurrent EM; in recurrent or persistent EM without a clear precipitant, consider work-up for solid organ or haematological malignancies.

KEY LEARNING POINTS

- Think widely about the causes of rashes in a systematic manner – is it viral, bacterial, immunological or medication-mediated?
- Screen patients with atypical infections for immunosuppressive disorder at presentation, such as HIV testing if readily available.
- The most commonly used severity score for Stevens–Johnson's syndrome (SJS) is the SCORTEN criteria.

A smashing Christmas

A 22-year-old woman with no past medical history accidentally slips on a wet paving stone on a nearby busy shopping street. She falls to her right and hits her jaw on a large concrete plant pot. She does not lose consciousness and remembers the whole event. She self-presents to the emergency department after being helped up by other pedestrians.

On examination, her observations are within normal limits and there is no cervical spine pain. On palpation of the face, she has tenderness across the entire mandible. You also note trismus, malocclusion and inability to open her mouth more than 3 finger breadths. Intra-orally, there is subtle early bruising at the gum line behind her right lower wisdom tooth and left first premolar. No teeth are loose. She has no other evidence of injury and there is no neurological deficit.

A CT scan of her facial bones is performed and is reported as normal. Due to ongoing pain and inability to open her mouth, the following radiograph is performed along with a PA mandible.

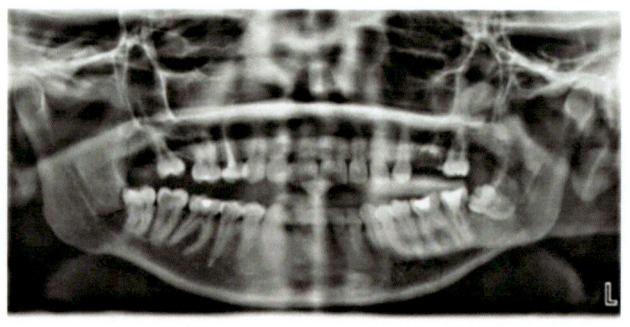 

1. What is the correct full name of the radiograph shown above?
   a. Orthopictogram
   b. Orthognathogram
   c. Orthopropogram
   d. Orthopantopogram
   e. Orthopantomogram

DOI: 10.1201/9781003461456-7

2. Which of the following abnormalities is NOT visualised on the radiograph?

    a. Impacted wisdom tooth

    b. Fracture through the right mandibular angle

    c. Fracture through the left mandibular body

    d. Periapical abscess

    e. Previous dental restorative work

3. How should this patient be managed, and what is the likely outcome?

    a. Discharge with analgesia and arrange urgent outpatient maxillofacial follow-up the next day

    b. Blood work-up, analgesia, NBM pending maxillofacial review, consider antibiotics, work-up for open reduction and internal fixation (ORIF)

    c. Blood work-up, analgesia, soft diet, oral antibiotics, conservative management

    d. Blood work-up, analgesia, NBM pending maxillofacial review, likely conservative management

    e. Blood work-up, analgesia, IV antibiotics, NBM pending maxillofacial review, likely conservative management

☑ 1e Orthopantomogram

This radiograph is called an orthopantomogram or OPG. It is useful for identifying subtle and undisplaced bony injuries of the mandible that can be missed by CT (as occurred in this case). It is taken standing or sitting, with the patient biting a radiolucent bite block to separate the jaw, which essentially makes the film weight-bearing. This exaggerates any bony deformities or displacement. The detector then swings from one side of the jaw to the other in an arc, creating a panoramic flat 2D image. It is difficult to capture completely in focus, as the radiograph detector must focus in-plane with a large number of structures from anterior to posterior. In this film, the anterior teeth are blurred as the detector was too posterior. Other pathologies imaged by this type of film include: temporomandibular joint (TMJ) issues including mandibular neck fractures; dental abscesses (look for a tear drop around the root); foreign bodies; and sometimes jaw dislocations.

☑ 2d Periapical abscess

There is a non-displaced fracture of the right mandibular angle (extending to the base of the lower right 8 [LR8] crown) with a further non-displaced left mandibular body fracture at lower left 5/6. The mandible is described as a 'half-polo-mint' and rarely breaks in just one location unless this is in the midline. Therefore, if one fracture is visualised, look for a second. The film also shows previous evidence of dental restorative work, including root canal treatment of upper right 4 (UR4) and lower left 7 (LL7). Upper left 5 (UL5) is carious with a partially fractured crown. Having a basic understanding of dentition is important for all healthcare professionals. In humans, dentition is described as primary (baby or milk teeth, 20 in total: 8 incisors, 4 canines and 8 molars) or permanent (adult teeth, 32 in total: 8 incisors, 4 canines, 8 premolars and 12 molars). Alpha-numeric notation designates the quadrant and tooth position from the midline; permanent teeth are numbered 1 to 8 whilst primary teeth are represented by letters A to E, with the prefixes designating the laterality and upper or lower jaw: L (left), R (right), U (upper), L (lower). When examining dental radiographs, dental caries appear as a radiolucent defect in the enamel whilst radiolucency at the apex is caused by a periapical (dental) abscess.

☑ 3b Blood work-up, analgesia, NBM pending maxillofacial review, consider antibiotics, work-up for ORIF

There are two important learning points from this case. Firstly, bilateral mandibular fractures such as this are rarely stable and generally cannot be managed conservatively; the clinical presentation of trismus, reduced mouth opening and malocclusion should herald suspicion of an unstable fracture caused by pulling on the fragment by the pterygoids. Secondly, the involvement of the dental root means that this should be treated as an open fracture. Broad-spectrum antibiotics and anaerobic cover are indicated to cover human oral microbiota according to local microbiology guidelines (for example, co-amoxiclav). This patient would therefore not be suitable for discharge and was referred to the on-call maxillofacial surgical team for ORIF. Mandibular fractures are the second most common facial fractures after nasal and are most often seen in young males, frequently caused by direct trauma from physical assault. Most mandibular fractures do not require emergency intervention, but it is vital to remember to exclude any other traumatic injuries. During assessment, ensure to assess for asymmetry, deformity, external or internal swelling/haematoma and malocclusion; test sensation to lower lip and chin (associated risk of damage to inferior alveolar nerve); and look for evidence of an open fracture.

KEY LEARNING POINTS

- The clinical signs of trismus, reduced mouth opening and malocclusion strongly suggest a clinical mandibular fracture.
- An orthopantomogram radiograph is a useful diagnostic tool even when CT is available as it is effectively a load-bearing image making undisplaced fractures more prominent and easier to identify.
- Look carefully for a second point of fracture in a mandible due to the half-polo-mint structure meaning that isolated single-point fractures are very rare.

Abdominal pain and distension in a child

A 7-year-old boy presents to the emergency department (ED) with his parents. They describe a 3-day history of generalised abdominal pain with associated distension, diarrhoea and vomiting. He has opened his bowels around 5 times today. It is described as loose but not explosive or bloody. He vomited after eating this morning; this was not projectile, contained foodstuffs and was not faeculent.

His parents inform you he was diagnosed with Hirschsprung's disease at birth and had surgery as a baby, but they are unsure of the exact procedure.

On examination, the child appears uncomfortable but is not restless or irritable. Observations are within normal limits for his age. His abdomen is distended, tympanic to percussion and generally tender with no focal areas and no rebound tenderness present.

An abdominal radiograph is performed.

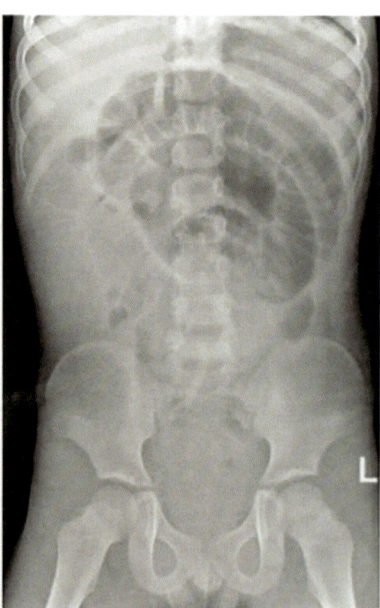

DOI: 10.1201/9781003461456-8

1. Though not necessarily present in this patient, which one of the following is a life-threatening complication of Hirschsprung's disease (HD) that you must consider in the ED?

   a. Colonic volvulus

   b. Gastroenteritis

   c. Intestinal obstruction

   d. Hirschsprung-associated enterocolitis

   e. Overflow diarrhoea

2. Which of the following is INCORRECT regarding HD?

   a. The prevalence is greater in females compared to males

   b. Normally both the small and large bowel are affected

   c. It is a motor disorder of the gastrointestinal tract

   d. The gold standard diagnostic test is an intestinal biopsy

   e. There is an absence of ganglion cells in the bowel wall

3. Which of the following are potential causes of distal intestinal obstruction in infants?

   a. Meconium ileus

   b. Intestinal atresia

   c. Meconium plug syndrome

   d. Anorectal malformation

   e. All of the above

☑ 1d Hirschsprung-associated enterocolitis

The abdominal radiograph in this patient confirms a diagnosis of small bowel obstruction with centrally lying bowel loops with clear demonstration of valvulae conniventes. In this patient, the cause is likely to be recurrent adhesional obstruction secondary to the original operation. Management should be to pass an NG tube to decompress the stomach and careful replacement of fluids and electrolytes. This patient should receive prompt surgical assessment to consider possible operative options such as laparotomy or adhesiolysis. Thinking slightly wider about untreated HD, the most serious complication is Hirschsprung-associated enterocolitis (HAEC). This is an inflammatory disorder of the colon in children with HD, commonly associated with complete or partial bowel obstruction. It is the most common cause of significant morbidity and mortality in children with HD. It can occur before and/or after pull-through surgery and is more common in <2 years of age, undiagnosed HD, trisomy 21 and long-segment HD. Diagnosis is clinical, based on symptoms and signs such as explosive and foul-smelling diarrhoea which may be bloody, vomiting, reduced oral intake, fever, lethargy, abdominal pain and distension. Mild cases may be misdiagnosed as gastroenteritis. Severe cases may display haemodynamic instability and peritonitis. Abdominal radiographs should be performed which would show dilated bowel loops, pneumatosis and a 'cut-off sign' in the rectosigmoid; this is gaseous distension of the proximal colon followed by absence of gas in distal colon. Management should include fluid resuscitation for shock or hypovolaemia, broad-spectrum IV antibiotics to cover aerobic and anaerobic organisms, and urgent surgical review. The other provided diagnoses should be considered in HD, and in particular volvulus or obstruction can also be a cause of morbidity and mortality, but HAEC should not be forgotten in these patients.

☑ 2b Normally both the small and large bowel are affected

HD is the main genetic cause of intestinal obstruction characterised by the absence of intramural parasympathetic ganglia of the myenteric and submucosal plexuses of the colon and rectum and does not affect the small bowel. It is classified as a neurocristopathy as it involves the neural crest. Individuals tend to have mutations in several genes that predispose them to developing HD. The absence of the ganglia leads to lack of normal gut peristalsis, leading to collection of stool in the large bowel, which can eventually lead to bowel obstruction. It is usually diagnosed in the neonatal period due to failure to pass meconium, abdominal distension, vomiting or neonatal enterocolitis. Some are not diagnosed until infancy or childhood, when they present with severe constipation, chronic abdominal distension and vomiting. Diagnosis is made by rectal biopsy using histochemical staining for acetylcholinesterase. HD is an isolated trait in many cases, but can be associated with chromosomal abnormalities, such as trisomy 21.

☑ 3e All of the above

Signs of bowel obstruction in neonates and infants, alongside those described above, include bile-stained vomiting (never ignore in a newborn), increased gastric residuals before feeding and absent or decreased bowel sounds. Atresia can affect the duodenum or jejunoileum. Duodenal atresia occurs due to a lesion at the level of the papilla of Vater (the second part of the duodenum), is associated with trisomy 21 in 25% of cases, and radiographs show a characteristic 'double-bubble' appearance. Jejunoileal atresia can occur anywhere along the small bowel, with radiographs showing air-fluid levels proximal to the lesion. Meconium ileus occurs due to thick meconium in the bowel leading to obstruction and ileus. Approximately 90% of these patients have cystic fibrosis. Abdominal radiographs may show the 'ground-glass' sign due to meconium mixed with swallowed air. Meconium plug syndrome is the most common cause of distal intestinal obstruction and can be diagnosed with a contrast enema before abdominal radiograph. The enema is often therapeutic, allowing plugs to be extruded and normal bowel function to resume. Anorectal malformations can vary in severity and terminology also depends on the gender of the child. They range from imperforate anus to perineal fistulae, fistulae to urethra, prostate, bladder neck or vaginal vestibule.

KEY LEARNING POINTS

- Hirschsprung's disease can be associated with multiple complications both before and after corrective surgery, and even with mild symptoms do not forget to consider Hirschsprung-associated enterocolitis.
- Hirschsprung's disease is due to multiple genetic mutations but is strongly associated with some other chromosomal abnormalities, such as trisomy 21.
- Never ignore bilious vomiting in any patient. It signifies a proximal bowel obstruction and will warrant a surgical opinion.

CASE 9

Abdominal pain in a heatwave

A 43-year-old Bengali-speaking man is brought in by ambulance after his wife found him collapsed at home; he reportedly was confused and disorientated, slumped in a chair on their balcony. The confusion self-resolved after 1 minute. During the past week, he has been complaining of lower back and abdominal pain and feeling feverish, and he describes having poor oral water intake in the recent heatwave. Past medical history includes duodenal perforation leading to a laparotomy in 2019 and renal stones.

His initial observations are recorded as HR 98, BP 101/78, SpO$_2$ 98% on room air, RR 20, temperature 38.2°C (100.7°F) and GCS 15/15. On examination, he is warm and clammy to touch, chest clear to auscultation, the abdomen is soft, but there is generalised tenderness throughout.

There are no neurological signs on examination.

1. What is your initial management plan?
    a. Draw bloods (FBC/U&Es/CRP/coagulation profile), urine culture, 500 mL crystalloid fluid bolus
    b. Draw bloods (FBC/U&Es/CRP/coagulation profile), blood cultures, urine culture, 500 mL crystalloid fluid bolus, IV antibiotics
    c. Draw bloods (FBC/U&Es/CRP), blood cultures, urine culture, 500 mL crystalloid fluid bolus
    d. Draw bloods (FBC/U&Es/CRP), urine dipstick, 500 mL crystalloid fluid bolus, IV antibiotics
    e. Draw bloods (FBC/U&Es/CRP/coagulation profile), group & screen, urine dipstick, 500 mL crystalloid fluid bolus, IV antibiotics

You receive a call from the biochemistry lab due to an acute kidney injury (AKI) warning:

   Cr 160 (previously 90), eGFR 43 (previously 84), Urea 6.6

You review the remaining bloods and note a CRP 131, WCC 19.8, neuts 15.

Urine dipstick: positive for blood (3+), leucocytes (2+) and nitrites (2+).

DOI: 10.1201/9781003461456-9

A non-contrast CT KUB is performed, and the coronal view is shown.

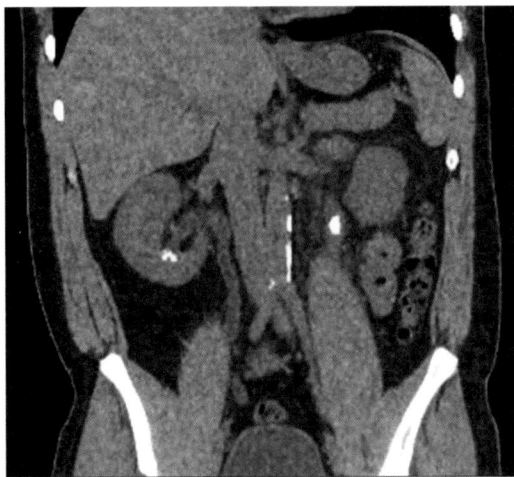

2. What is evident on the images that could account for the patient's presentation and blood results?

    a. Bilateral calyceal stones with a large obstructing calculus in the left proximal ureter with hydronephrosis

    b. Bilateral calyceal stones with mild bilateral hydronephrosis

    c. Large calculus in the left VUJ and bilateral calyceal stones

    d. Bilateral calyceal stones with a large obstructing calculus in the right proximal ureter

    e. Thickened appendix, evidence of mesenteric fat stranding and free fluid in the pelvis

3. Which of the following is the most common composition of urolithiasis?

    a. Calcium phosphate

    b. Urate

    c. Struvite

    d. Cysteine

    e. Calcium oxalate

☑ **1b Draw bloods (FBC/U&Es/CRP/coagulation profile), blood cultures, urine culture, 500 mL crystalloid fluid bolus, IV antibiotics**

The history is somewhat vague, though we can identify this patient has had a transient loss of consciousness (TLOC) and appears to have an infection on board (borderline tachycardia, hypotension from likely baseline and history of fevers). He warrants a full work-up with regard to possible sepsis, i.e. full blood work-up including blood cultures. Additionally, given the history of renal stones and abdominal pain, a urine culture should be sent. In terms of initial management, IV fluid resuscitation and IV antibiotics according to local microbiology guidelines (for example, 1.5 g cefuroxime) should be commenced promptly since there are reasonable clinical grounds to suggest an ascending UTI with lower back pain and fever. Additional measures, not included here, would also be to complete a full assessment for TLOC, including ECG, lying and standing BP and full neurological assessment. When thinking of the causes of syncope ask yourself, 'Is it the box (brain), the pump (heart) or the wiring (nerves or blood vessels)?'

☑ **2a Bilateral calyceal stones with a large obstructing calculus in the left proximal ureter with hydronephrosis**

Seen best in the accompanying video, this non-contrast CT KUB shows a large urinary calculus (8.5 mm) in the left proximal ureter, just after the pelvi-ureteric junction (PUJ), with a smaller one (3.5 mm) lying superiorly. This is associated with mild hydronephrosis and perinephric fat stranding, which is suggestive of co-existing infection. In addition, there is a high stone burden with multiple bilateral calyceal stones, with some of these resembling staghorn calculi. The most likely cause of the patient's blood results (AKI and marked inflammatory response) is an obstructing stone with associated infection, which is a true urological emergency. This patient should be resuscitated according to SEPSIS 6 guidelines and referred promptly to the urologists for admission and definitive surgical management. It was felt that the collapse/reduced consciousness that drove the patient's presentation was a possible vasovagal secondary to poor oral intake in hot weather, associated with increased insensible losses due to fevers. In addition, hot weather is known to precipitate formation of renal stones and thereby increasing the risk of obstructive urolithiasis. With such a high stone burden, this patient should be screened for genetic or enzymic causes as well as dietary triggers.

☑ **3e Calcium oxalate**

Stone composition varies widely depending on metabolic alterations, geography and presence of infection. The commonest composition of urolithiasis is calcium oxalate +/– phosphate (~75%), followed by struvite (15%), pure calcium phosphate (7–9%), uric acid (5–8%), cystine (1%), other (1%). Stones can also have mixed composition.

Additional blood tests which aid the urologists with the reason for stone formation include serum urate and bone profile (calcium and phosphate). Ninety-nine percent of stones are visible on non-contrast CT, hence why this is investigation of choice. In comparison ultrasound has a sensitivity of 24%, and only calcium stones are radio-opaque on radiographs. Indications for surgical management include: larger stones (typically >5 mm), extended duration of symptoms, proximal stones, infection or sepsis, solitary kidney or failed conservative management. Retrograde ureteric stent insertion is first line, unless acute sepsis as in this case or another reason makes the patient unsuitable for anaesthetic. Other options include percutaneous nephrostomy with or without antegrade stent insertion for patients with difficult retrograde access or abnormal anatomy, or extracorporeal shock wave lithotripsy for patients who are unsuitable for invasive management. In this patient, the ideal treatment is to treat sepsis and perform a percutaneous nephrostomy to allow renal function to recover. Once the infection has cleared, then stent insertion or surgical stone excision can be considered.

KEY LEARNING POINTS

- When assessing the patient who has presented with a collapse, think widely about causes in a structured manner as the loss of consciousness is usually the endpoint of another underlying cause.
- The presence of active infection is a relative contraindication to ureteric stent insertion.
- Screening for genetic and dietary causes of renal stones should be performed in patients with recurrent renal stones or high stone burden via specialist outpatient services.

Abnormal blood gas

A 62-year-old woman presents due to generalised weakness for the past 2 days. She has a history of endometrial cancer and underwent radical chemotherapy several months ago. Over the past 2–3 weeks, she has noted increasing swelling of her lower limbs and describes increasingly itchy skin.

Initial observations are recorded as HR 97, BP 221/93, SpO_2 100% on room air, RR 24, temperature 37.3°C (99.4 °F) and GCS 15/15.

She has difficult venous access, and you assist by performing ultrasound guided cannulation into a reasonably sized deep vein.

On the venous blood gas (VBG), you note some abnormal results.

Component	Value	Flag	Ref Range	Units	Status
Source	Venous				Final
pH	7.364				Final
Carbon Dioxide Partial Pressure	5.04			kPa	Final
Oxygen Partial Pressure	11.8			kPa	Final
Potassium	8.8	∧		mmol/L	Final
Comment:					
Value above reference range					
Sodium	136			mmol/L	Final
Ionised Calcium	1.12	∨		mmol/L	Final
Comment:					
Value below reference range					
Chloride	103			mmol/L	Final
Glucose	3.5			mmol/L	Final
Lactate	1.1			mmol/L	Final
Urea	20.3	∧		mmol/L	Final
Comment:					
Value above reference range					
Total Haemoglobin	83	∨		g/l	Final
Comment:					
Value below reference range					
Deoxyhaemoglobin	2.5			%	Final
Oxyhaemoglobin	95.5			%	Final
Saturated Oxygen	97.4			%	Final
Carboxyhaemoglobin	0.9			%	Final
Methaemoglobin	1.1			%	Final
Bilirubin	9			micromol/l	Final
Standard Base Excess	-3.9	∨		mmol/L	Final
Standard Bicarbonate	21.4			mmol/L	Final

DOI: 10.1201/9781003461456-10

1. What is the next most appropriate step in management?

   a. Administer 5 mg salbutamol via nebuliser

   b. Administer 10 mL 10% calcium gluconate IV over 5 minutes

   c. Administer 10 mL 10% calcium chloride IV over 5 minutes

   d. Administer 10 units actrapid in 250 mL 10% glucose IV over 15 minutes

   e. Administer 40 mg furosemide IV over 2 minutes

A 12-lead ECG is performed.

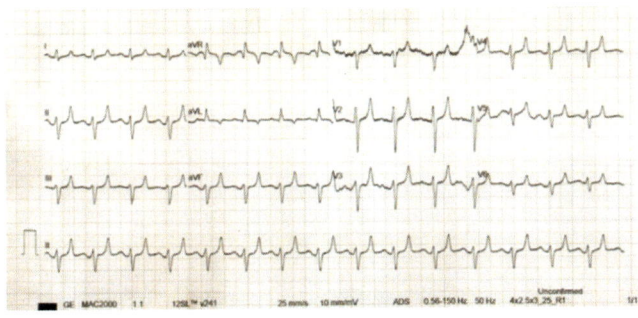 

2. Which one of the following is present in this ECG?

   a. Prolonged PR interval

   b. Tall, tented T waves

   c. Left bundle branch block

   d. Benign early repolarisation

   e. Right bundle branch block

3. Which of the following is NOT an indication for emergency haemofiltration?

   a. Uraemic encephalopathy

   b. Severe metabolic acidosis

   c. Refractory pulmonary oedema

   d. Hypercalcaemia

   e. Hyperthermia

☑ 1c Administer 10 mL of 10% calcium chloride IV over 5 minutes

The striking abnormality on this VBG is the potassium of 8.8 mmol/L. Whilst lowering this patient's potassium is a priority, it is most important in the first instance to give either calcium chloride or gluconate as a cardiac stabilising treatment. This should be given if the ECG shows any features of hyperkalaemia or if the potassium is over 6.5. Calcium chloride contains three times as much elemental calcium ions compared to gluconate and can be given as a bolus but may result in local thrombophlebitis. The correct dose of calcium chloride is 10 mL of 10% of calcium chloride over 5 minutes, whereas the correct dose of calcium gluconate is 30 mL of 10% calcium gluconate over 15 minutes. All of the other treatments are indicated in acute potassium-lowering therapy but should be given once cardiac stabilising treatment has been given, especially in very high potassium levels as in this case.

☑ 2b Tall, tented T waves

The correct answer is the presence of tall, tented T waves. ECG changes in hyperkalaemia are progressive and directly linked to the serum potassium level. Changes typically appear first at 6.5 mmol/L whereby the atria are progressively paralysed. This results in flat and wide P waves, PR prolongation, and eventually totally absent P waves. The next threshold is at 7.0 mmol/L with delayed conduction and bradyarrhythmias (wide QRS, bundle branch block, high-grade AV block, sinus bradycardia, sine wave). Above 9.0 mmol/L you will typically see cardiac arrest with VF, pulseless electrical activity (PEA) with wide complexes or asystole.

This patient's relatively few ECG changes suggest that the hyperkalaemia is chronic and this apparent 'tolerance' to hyperkalaemia is typically seen in renal patients. This patient's creatinine came back at 1145 umol/L and subsequent imaging with CT showed post-renal obstruction due to progression of the endometrial cancer.

☑ 3d Hypercalcaemia

Haemofiltration is a form of renal replacement therapy (RRT) used in the critical care setting, where blood is pumped through an extracorporeal system that incorporates a semi-permeable membrane. Hydrostatic pressure on the blood side of the membrane (or filter) causes plasma water to be pushed across it, termed ultrafiltration, and small molecules (<50 000 Daltons) are 'dragged' across the membrane with the water by convection. The ultrafiltrate is then discarded and replacement fluid is added depending on the desired fluid balance. This differs from haemodialysis where solutes move across the semi-permeable membrane along their concentration gradient by diffusion. This means molecules can move from blood to dialysate (for example, urea and potassium), or vice versa (for example, bicarbonate). The main indications for RRT are: acute kidney injury (AKI) with hyperkalaemia (where medical management is insufficient); symptomatic uraemia (i.e. pruritus, nausea, encephalopathy or pericarditis); fluid overload (not responding to diuretics); severe metabolic acidosis; or the removal of certain drugs (for example, lithium, salicylates, methanol, ethylene glycol). In terms of when to start RRT, this should be prompted by the patient's general condition and rate of change of the above parameters rather than set arbitrary numbers. Hypercalcaemia alone is not an indication for RRT.

KEY LEARNING POINTS

- ECG changes in hyperkalaemia are progressive and linked to the degree of hyperkalaemia but may be attenuated or absent in chronically elevated cases such as renal patients.
- Calcium chloride is the preferred agent in the treatment of acute hyperkalaemia as it has approximately three times the free elemental calcium compared to the gluconate compound.
- Renal replacement therapy should be considered in cases whereby medical therapy alone is not sufficient or there is symptomatic uraemia, metabolic acidosis or fluid overload.

CASE 11

An elderly patient on warfarin

An 88-year-old woman is brought in by ambulance to the emergency department (ED) after her neighbour called the emergency services as she appeared confused and not quite herself. On arrival in the department, she is speaking coherently but is disorientated to time and place. She complains of a moderate headache but finds it difficult to describe its features. However, she denies sustaining any recent falls.

Her past medical history includes atrial fibrillation, for which she is anticoagulated with warfarin, and chronic kidney disease stage 3.

On assessment in the triage area, you note initial observations of HR 100, BP 179/90, SpO$_2$ 97% on room air, GCS 14/15, temperature 36.3°C (97.3°F). Focused neurological examination is grossly normal.

1. Which of the following is the best immediate management?
   a. Oral analgesia, ECG, urine dip, redirect to urgent treatment centre for GP review
   b. Draw bloods (FBC/U&Es/INR), ECG, urine dip, stream to majors
   c. Draw bloods (FBC/U&Es/INR), ECG, urine dip, 10 mg amlodipine, stream to majors
   d. Draw bloods (FBC/U&Es/INR), ECG, urine dip, 5 mg amlodipine, stream to majors
   e. Draw bloods (FBC/U&Es/INR), ECG, urine dip, move to resuscitation room for immediate blood pressure control with IV labetalol infusion

A non-contrast CT head is performed.

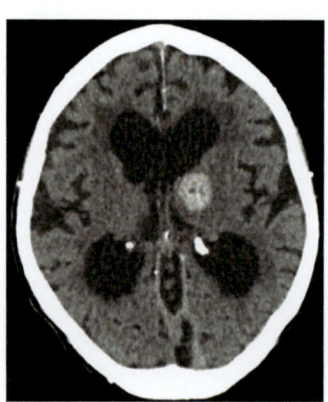 

DOI: 10.1201/9781003461456-11

2. Which of the following is the best description of the findings?

   a. Haemorrhagic intracranial metastatic malignancy

   b. Infected acute epidermoid cyst

   c. Bilateral acute hypertensive haemorrhages

   d. Bilateral calcifying oligodendroglioma

   e. Giant intracerebral aneurysm

You review the blood results and note INR 4.5 and eGFR 15.

On reassessment, the patient's GCS is still 14/15 but she complains of an ongoing headache despite analgesia. You move the patient to the resuscitation room for close observation including blood pressure monitoring and neurological observations every 15 minutes and refer her to the stroke specialist team.

3. Which of the following is the best treatment option?

   a. Dexamethasone 8 mg IV

   b. Vitamin K 10 mg IV

   c. Amlodipine 10 mg PO

   d. Vitamin K 10 mg IV and prothrombin complex concentrate (Octaplex)

   e. Vitamin K 10 mg IV and fresh frozen plasma

☑ 1b Draw bloods (FBC/U&Es/INR), ECG, urine dip, stream to majors

This vague presentation of an elderly confused patient will be familiar to many who have worked in the ED and there is a wide range of differential diagnoses at this stage (think of your surgical sieve). There are a few features that warrant further investigation and thorough assessment by an emergency medicine practitioner; her age, presence of a headache, hypertension and warfarin use hopefully raise alarms that she is at increased risk of potential intracranial pathology, and therefore redirection to the urgent treatment centre is inappropriate. With the current blood pressure recording and no sign of acute progressive target organ damage, this is currently not a hypertensive emergency and there is no immediate requirement to administer antihypertensives. Additionally, with oral amlodipine there is a potential risk of lowering the blood pressure too quickly, which in turn can compromise perfusion to vital organs (including the brain) where autoregulatory mechanisms cannot compensate. Therefore, for hypertensive emergencies, controlled and progressive reductions in blood pressure are typically achieved by IV short-acting antihypertensives such as labetalol, aiming to reduce the mean arterial pressure (MAP) by up to 25% within the first hour. The administration of these IV short-acting antihypertensives requires continuous observation and monitoring, as well as admission to a high dependency or intensive care setting.

☑ 2c Bilateral acute hypertensive haemorrhages

The CT clip shows multiple bilateral hyperdensities, including a large focus in the left thalamus, which in the context of this patient are likely to represent acute hypertensive haemorrhages. A haemorrhagic metastatic deposit could still be a possibility and careful clinical evaluation for a primary, combined with either a CT head with contrast or MRI, would help to differentiate this. Hypertensive intracerebral haemorrhages are most commonly seen in the basal ganglia, thalamus, pons or cerebellum. Depending on the location, the patient may have specific neurological features, such as downward deviation of eyes and lack of pupillary response in thalamic haemorrhage or posterior circulation symptoms of vertigo, ataxia, nausea and vomiting in cerebellar haemorrhage. Note there is also pronounced dilation of lateral ventricles – this could represent acute hydrocephalus if combined with dilated 3rd and 4th ventricles and this CT should be compared to previous imaging if available as well a good clinical neurological examination, including assessment for papilloedema.

☑ 3d Vitamin K 10 mg IV and prothrombin complex concentrate (Octaplex)

This patient has ongoing headache, significant hypertension, an INR of >4 and a CT scan suggestive of acute bleeding. Any patient on warfarin with major bleeding should be treated with IV vitamin K, and dried prothrombin complex concentrate (for example, 'Octaplex' or 'Beriplex'), which contains factors II, VII, IX and X. The dose is typically 25–50 units/kilogram, rounded to the nearest 500 units, and the maximum dose is 5000 units. Note that dried prothrombin complex concentrate requires authorisation by the on-call haematologist in some hospitals although it is best practice to consult them in any instances of high INR with bleeding. Repeat clotting profile should be sent 15 minutes after its administration and again at 4–6 hours if adequate correction is observed. Fresh frozen plasma can be used if dried prothrombin complex concentrate is unavailable, but again this should be with the involvement of the haematologists. Stroke specialists manage the majority of spontaneous hypertensive bleeds with haematology input and involvement of neurosurgeons if necessary (needing external ventricular drain, EVD) insertion, decompressive craniectomy, associated aneurysmal bleeds). In terms of blood pressure management, this needs to be determined as a balance of benefits versus risk. In this case, the patient was managed with an intravenous labetalol infusion (target systolic BP 140–150 mmHg). If hypertensive intracranial haemorrhage is associated with raised ICP, cerebral perfusion may be impaired with reduced MAP so cautious reduction is advised.

KEY LEARNING POINTS

- Assessment of the older confused patient requires a careful approach combining judicious history-taking, examination and targeted investigations.
- Have a low threshold for cranial imaging in patients on anticoagulation and confusion or neurological signs.
- Liaise early with haematologists for specialist advice regarding reversal of anticoagulation especially in the context of intracranial bleeding.
- Blood pressure management in patients with intracranial haemorrhage is probably best managed in at least an HDU setting with an arterial line and intravenous agents.

An unusual ECG

A 36-year-old woman presents to the emergency department with severe generalised abdominal pain with vomiting immediately after eating or drinking. She states she is unable to keep any food or oral fluids down and is feeling dehydrated. She has not eaten anything from a restaurant or takeaway and has no unwell contacts. She describes having had multiple similar episodes in the past and was treated at a specialist medical unit but cannot remember the medical diagnosis. She takes no regular medications currently and has no known allergies.

An ECG is performed as part of the work-up, and you note an abnormality.

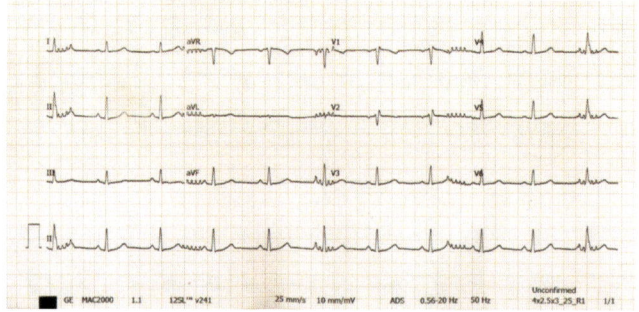 

1. Which of the following best describes what the ECG shows?

    a. Intermittent atrial flutter

    b. Cardiac pacemaker rhythm

    c. Mobitz type I AV block (Wenkebach)

    d. Intermittent atrial fibrillation

    e. Intermittent artefact or interference

DOI: 10.1201/9781003461456-12

2.   What is the likely origin of the abnormality on this ECG?

   a.   Malfunction of cardiac pacemaker

   b.   ECG lead placement issue

   c.   Extra-cardiac electrical interference

   d.   Movement artefact, for example shivering

   e.   Electrolyte disturbance

The patient remembers that she had a medical procedure at a specialist unit, and you think this could be related to the observed ECG changes, but she is vague about the indications and specific details.

3.   What is the likely origin of the electrical abnormality in this instance?

   a.   Gastric pacemaker

   b.   Sacral nerve stimulator

   c.   Runaway pacemaker

   d.   Smartwatch

   e.   Deep brain stimulator (DBS)

☑ 1e Intermittent artefact or interference

Looking at the RR interval, one can see that this patient has regular heart rate with preceding P waves, which would rule out atrial fibrillation, which would be associated with an irregularly irregular rhythm and lack of P waves. Atrial flutter waves are typically regular at a rate of around 300 beats per minute with a 'saw-tooth' pattern best seen in leads II, III and aVF, therefore this option can also be excluded. The abnormal waves are dissociated from and unrelated to the cardiac cycle, they are not related to the patient's native P waves and they have no effect on QRS complexes when they fall together. The native P waves and QRS complexes can be seen superimposed on top of the arte-factual waves (as seen in complexes 6 and 11 on the lead II rhythm strip). In between the abnormality, native P waves precede QRS with no change in PR interval, excluding Mobitz type I. Putting all this together, we can conclude abnormal waves are likely to be interference i.e. artefact.

☑ 2c Extra-cardiac electrical interference

A cardiac pacemaker malfunction is very unlikely to present in this way. Pacemaker malfunctions may be due to problems with sensing or pacing. Sensing issues are due to undersensing or oversensing; undersensing is where the pacemaker fails to sense native activity resulting in asynchronous pacing, whereas oversensing is where electrical signals are inappropriately recognised as native cardiac activity and pacing is inhibited. Pacing issues are due to output failure when a paced stimulus is not produced where expected, or failure to capture when a paced stimulus does not lead to myocardial depo-larisation. These could be seen as rapid ventricular pacing if oversensing or continuous spikes if runaway pacing. Both would be associated with the cardiac cycle and therefore not likely to be the cause of the above abnormality. Extra-cardiac lead displacement of a pacemaker is very unlikely, and even then, as with the above, it would not produce multiple consistent short amplitude waveforms like this. ECG lead placement would not cause such regular artefact. The regularity of the intervals, the identical amplitude and spacing of the waves and consistent 5 regular waveforms mean this could not simply be movement artefact or human movement and would have to be some other extra-cardiac regular electrical interference.

☑ 3a Gastric pacemaker

As is alluded to in the brief history, this woman has had a history of recurrent episodes of abdominal pain and vomiting requiring hospital attendances. It transpired she had a past history of gastroparesis for which she has an implanted gastric pacemaker. This involves two bipolar leads that are inserted into the walls of the stomach and a pulse generator in the upper abdomen, both in close proximity to the heart. Typically, the stimulation is high-frequency (14 Hz) and low-energy stimulation, which is programmed by a physician. Here we can see this stimulation produces repetitive low amplitude signals of five beats.

There are other implantable stimulating devices or 'extra-cardiac pacemakers' which have multiple clinical indications, including DBS for Parkinson's disease and other dystonias, spinal cord stimulators for refractory back pain or migraine, sacral nerve neuro-modulators for urinary incontinence or urgency, and many others. The devices vary in type of lead, output amplitude, pulse width, frequency and cycle. Any of these have the potential to cause internal artefact to the ECG trace. A careful history and clinical examination should give sufficient clues to the type of implanted device as well as any implantable medical devices visualised on radiographs.

KEY LEARNING POINTS

- A systemised approach to ECG interpretation is key to successful identification of abnormalities.
- Extra-cardiac electrical interference may occur from a variety of devices placed near the heart.
- History, clinical examination for masses (boxes), scar location and simple radiography may be useful adjuncts to determining device type in cases where the patient cannot recall the exact device type.

CASE 13

Assault

A 63-year-old man self-presents to the emergency department after being assaulted in a nearby bar. He describes receiving a blow to the left side of his face but is unsure if the assailant used a weapon or fist. He reports that immediately after the assault he experienced blurred vision, which resolved within a few minutes. He denies losing consciousness, does not feel confused, has not vomited, has not noticed any fluid coming from his nose or ears, and denies any focal neurological symptoms. He does not have any neck pain. His main complaint is ongoing facial pain, mild headache and swelling around his left eye.

He is fit and well and has no regular medications.

On initial assessment, all observations are within normal limits. Primary survey is unremarkable apart from left-sided periorbital ecchymosis with a large haematoma over the upper eyelid, subconjunctival haemorrhage and proptosis. Visual acuity is normal, movement of the globe is normal and the remainder of the cranial nerve examination is unremarkable.

1. Which of the following imaging investigations would you request next?
   a. CT cervical spine
   b. CT facial bones
   c. CT head with contrast
   d. CT head and facial bones
   e. CT polytrauma

DOI: 10.1201/9781003461456-13

CT imaging is performed and while waiting for the report, the nursing team notifies you that the patient is complaining of increased eye pain and new diplopia.

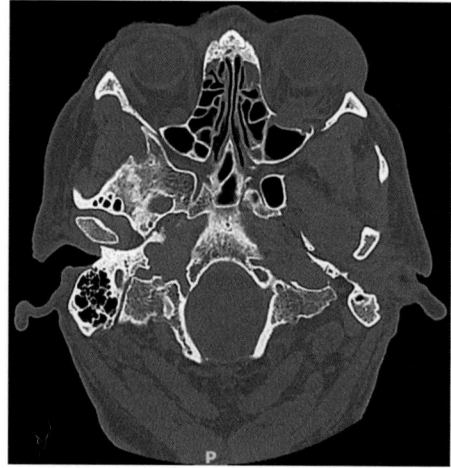

You review the scans with a senior colleague.

2. Which of the following findings on the scan are you most concerned about?
    a. Orbital cellulitis
    b. Retrobulbar haemorrhage
    c. Pre-septal cellulitis
    d. Lateral maxillary sinus fracture
    e. Orbital floor fracture

The patient is moved to the resuscitation room and the attending registrar prepares to perform a lateral canthotomy under local anaesthetic.

3. Which of the following statements about the lateral canthotomy is correct?
    a. Point the needle towards the globe when injecting local lidocaine with 1:80 000 adrenaline
    b. The inferior crus of the lateral canthus tendon should be incised
    c. There is danger of dividing the tear duct, which must be identified and protected prior to division
    d. The superior crus of the lateral canthus tendon should be incised
    e. Tarsal eversion of the superior eyelid must be performed first

☑   1d CT head and facial bones

In the investigation of facial trauma, various CT scans with specific protocols may be utilised to comprehensively assess different aspects of the facial structures. The choice of CT scans depends on the suspected injuries and the clinical presentation. This patient has sustained an obvious facial trauma, and bones of the orbit are at risk of fracture with the pattern of injury in this case. Along with the orbit, this will also assess for fractures of nasal bones, maxilla and mandible. Patients with facial fractures are at high risk of intracranial injury and therefore a CT head should also be performed. The history and examination findings are not concerning for c-spine injury, and therefore CT C-spine is not indicated in this case; however, if there is any suggestion of c-spine tenderness, or the patient is difficult to assess due to intoxication, have a low threshold to image the c-spine to exclude potentially catastrophic injury. Clinical decision-making tools such as the NEXUS criteria can be used to clinical assess and clear the cervical spine in a standardised manner. Considering the other options, a CT head alone will not provide adequate coverage of the facial bones and so is inadequate, and a CT head with contrast is used to look for enhancing lesions such as tumours and again not indicated in this trauma case.

☑   2b Retrobulbar haemorrhage

The provided CT scan shows a bone window of the facial bones. The two gross abnormalities demonstrated are a left-sided orbital floor fracture and a retrobulbar haemorrhage. The orbital floor is displaced inferiorly, and you should appreciate the increased hyperdense matter posteriorly to the globe, which is 'pushing' the globe forwards; note the level of the anterior aspect of the left globe compared to the right. The retrobulbar space is enclosed by bone on its medial, lateral and posterior aspects, therefore any rise in pressure within this space (i.e. due to haemorrhage) will cause a forward shift of the globe, seen as proptosis clinically. Anterior displacement of the globe is limited by the medial and lateral canthal tendons, which act essentially as retaining straps. Continued forward motion will compress the globe, raising intraocular pressure, reducing blood flow to the retina and optic nerve, risking permanent sight-loss. This is an ophthalmic emergency, which requires urgent lateral canthotomy and cantholysis to decompress the orbit and preserve ocular function. Any visual disturbance, impaired extraocular motility, relative afferent pupillary defect (RAPD) or raised intraocular pressure (does the globe feel 'woody' compared to the unaffected side?) associated with suspected or confirmed retrobulbar haemorrhage should be assessed immediately and lateral canthotomy performed.

☑ 3b The inferior crus of the lateral canthus tendon should be incised

Lateral canthotomy and cantholysis is the treatment for orbital compartment syndrome, which involves surgically exposing the lateral canthal tendon and its inferior crus to relieve intraorbital pressure. The only contraindication is a patient with suspected open globe. This is suggested by corneal laceration, hyphema, herniated uveal tissue or a shallow anterior chamber. To perform the procedure, firstly gather equipment: sterile gloves, gown, drapes, gauze and position the patient supine with head raised 10–20 degrees, with eyelids and head stabilised. Prepare the area with antiseptic and drape. Inject 1–2 mL of local anaesthetic (for example, 1% lidocaine with 1:80 000 adrenaline) into the planned incision site, ensuring to direct tip of needle away from the globe. Horizontally clamp across the lateral canthus for approximately 1 minute with straight mosquito forceps to help with haemostasis and displace oedema for the incision. Then cut from the lateral canthus to the rim of the orbit using iris scissors. The full length of the incision is around 1–2 cm and should be no more than 2 cm to avoid the temporal branch of the facial nerve. Lift the lateral portion of the inferior eyelid, exposing the lateral canthal tendon and cut the inferior crus, ensuring that your scissors are pointing away from the globe. Curved iris scissors are preferred to straight ones in this regard as they will naturally point slightly inferiorly. Once performed successfully, the globe can expand out of the orbit thus relieving raised intraorbital pressure. Apply gentle pressure to the wound as required for haemostasis. Lateral canthotomy and cantholysis can be left to spontaneously granulate and heal or may be electively repaired at a later date. Topical chloramphenicol ointment should be applied several times per day to the wound to prevent infection.

KEY LEARNING POINTS

- Patients presenting with facial trauma are at high risk of associated intracranial injury and so CT head and facial bones is recommended.
- Lateral canthotomy is a sight-saving procedure and can be safely performed by non-ophthalmologists or facial surgeons after focused training.
- Remember to identify and cut the inferior crus of the lateral canthal tendon.
- Intra-ocular pressures can be measured pre and post to check the effectiveness of the procedure.

CASE 14

Blown pupil

You respond to a tannoy request to urgently assess a new patient in the resuscitation room.

You receive a 38-year-old female who is in police custody. The ambulance crew inform you that she had been seen at another hospital earlier in the day following an assault, but self-discharged prior to full assessment. The ambulance service was called by police as the patient became increasingly agitated and intermittently drowsy in custody. They report that she dropped her GCS from 14/15 to 8/15 during transfer to hospital and her right pupil has become dilated with a sluggish reaction to light in the last 10 minutes. She has external evidence of head injury but no other obvious injuries reported by the crew.

1. Which of the following is the best initial management plan?
   a. Place a trauma call, ABCDE assessment, insert 2 x 18 G cannulae, draw bloods (FBC/U&Es/coagulation profile), give cautious IV crystalloid fluids to support BP
   b. Place a trauma call, ABCDE assessment, apply high-flow oxygen, insert 2 x 18 G cannulae, draw bloods (FBC/U&Es/coagulation profile/group & screen), cautious IV fluids to support BP
   c. Fast bleep anaesthetist on-call, ABCDE assessment, prepare to sedate the patient to facilitate CT transfer
   d. Place a trauma call, ABCDE assessment, insert 2 x 18 G cannulae, draw bloods (FBC/U&Es/coagulation profile/group & screen), administer 2 litres IV crystalloid fluids stat
   e. ABCDE assessment, contact the local neurosurgery registrar on-call for advice

DOI: 10.1201/9781003461456-14

The anaesthetic team arrive promptly and intubate the patient whilst you arrange a CT head and cervical spine.

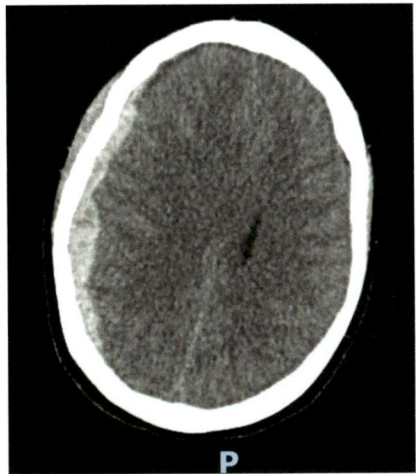

A colleague has gained collateral from the previous hospital and informs you the patient has a diagnosis of immune thrombocytopenic purpura (ITP) and her platelet count was 6 earlier that morning.

2. Which of the following is the next best management step?

   a. Administer 1 g tranexamic acid IV, request 2 pools of platelets immediately from the transfusion laboratory

   b. Administer andexanet alfa (Andexxa®) and 1 g tranexamic acid IV

   c. Activate the major haemorrhage protocol, transfuse the contents of the 'first pack'

   d. Administer 2 g tranexamic acid IV, request fresh frozen plasma (FFP) and cryopre-cipitate (CPP)

   e. Administer prothrombic concentrate complex (PCC) and 1 g tranexamic acid IV

3. Which anatomical location is usually the source of bleeding that leads to this pattern of injury?

   a. Middle meningeal artery

   b. Bridging veins

   c. Ruptured cortical veins

   d. Middle meningeal vein

   e. Temporal artery

☑ 1b Place a trauma call, ABCDE assessment, apply high-flow oxygen, insert 2 x 18 G cannulae, draw bloods (FBC/U&Es/ coagulation profile/group & screen), cautious IV fluids to support BP

In the context of trauma, the priority should always be the same: place a trauma call – this will bring people who can deal with Airway, Breathing, Circulation and Disability problems; a trauma team will typically include anaesthetic and/or intensive care unit teams, general surgeons, the orthopaedic team and emergency department (ED) nursing staff and/or critical care outreach nursing staff. The 'primary survey' is designed to assess the patient in an ABCDE fashion and be performed in under 5 minutes, and aims to identify and treat life-threatening injuries. A senior emergency medicine doctor usually leads the team. The low GCS and 'blown' pupil suggest an expanding intracranial mass, in this case likely to be blood. The blood compresses the brain causing uncal herniation, which compresses the 3rd cranial nerve and impairs the sympathetic fibres outflow, resulting in pupillary dilatation and anisocoria. This is not good news. This patient with her GCS currently at 8/15, in the absence of any other life-threatening injury, will need intubation and ventilation, not sedation, to prevent secondary brain injury and facilitate a safe transfer to CT and onward to a neurological centre if not found in your hospital. Don't forget to apply supplemental oxygen as per current ATLS guidelines.

☑ 2a Administer 1 g tranexamic acid IV, request 2 pools of platelets immediately from the transfusion laboratory

The CRASH-3 trial, published in 2019, provides evidence to support the use of tranexamic acid in traumatic intracranial haemorrhage; importantly, the earlier the tranexamic acid was given (<3 hours), the better the outcomes. Given the fact that tranexamic acid is readily available, cheap and was not associated with any increase in thromboembolic events in CRASH-3, it would be prudent to administer to patients with suspected/ confirmed traumatic intracranial haemorrhage, and patients with head injury and extracranial injury. In the case of severe bleeding in patients with a low platelet count, a platelet transfusion should be given as soon as possible. In some hospital Trusts the issuing of platelets must be authorised by a haematologist whereas others allow these to be requested without authorisation, so take time to familiarise yourself with local protocols where you are working. FFP and CPP contain differing constituents of clotting factors and fibrinogen; FFP tends to be used in multifactor deficiencies whereas CPP tends to be used when fibrinogen levels are low. Note that major haemorrhage protocols may also vary depending on where you work, and therefore again familiarise yourself with the protocols and what the blood bank provides in terms of 'packs' of blood components when these are activated. In general, pack 1 usually contains packed red cells (6 units) and FFP (4 units). Pack 2 normally contains 2 packs of CPP and one pool of platelets. In this patient, early recognition of the need for platelets will be key and a direct request is normally required as well as the assistance of a haematologist to guide correction.

☑ 3b Bridging veins

The CT scan shows an acute right-sided subdural haematoma with sulcal and ventricular effacement and midline shift. An acute subdural is usually the result of a tear in the wall of a bridging vein as it passes between the arachnoid and dural layers. As intracranial pressure (ICP) rises, blood is squeezed into dural venous sinuses, raising dural venous pressure causing more bleeding from the ruptured bridging veins. They stop growing when the pressure of the haematoma equalises with the ICP, as the space available for expansion shrinks. The middle meningeal artery injury is a common cause of extradural haemorrhage (seen as a lentiform shaped bleed), which is often seen as a result of trauma to the side of the head. Temporal artery bleeds are seen in superficial injuries, for example when a patient is 'bottled', and can bleed profusely. Their control may require suture ligation as simple pressure often fails. Bleeding from cortical veins could lead to subarachnoid haemorrhage.

KEY LEARNING POINTS

- The initial assessment management of trauma should follow ATLS guidelines no matter what scenario is presented as it allows one safe approach to identify and treat life-threatening injuries.
- Familiarise yourself with local major haemorrhage protocols and pack constituents as you may face scenarios needing additional products as part of the correction strategy.
- Subdural haematomas may present some hours after the initial injury as patients leak blood into the cranial cavity until the point of decompensation. This may be exacerbated by haematological conditions or medications.

CASE 15

Bradycardia

A 72-year-old man is brought in by ambulance complaining of severe 8/10 burning and aching central chest pain starting 3 hours previously with associated dizziness, sweating and nausea. He reports a past medical history of hypertension, benign prostatic hyperplasia and he mentions a previous 'irregular heart beat'.

The initial observations are recorded as HR 40, BP 176/88, RR 18, SpO$_2$ 98% on room air, 15/15 afebrile, GCS 15. The cardiorespiratory examination is unremarkable and there is no radio-radial or radio-femoral delay.

You note results of the initial venous blood gas (VBG) showing K$^+$ 2.8, otherwise no other abnormalities are detected.

An ECG is performed.

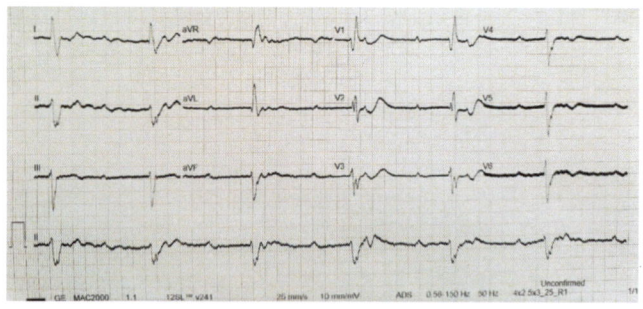 

1. Which of the following is the best interpretation of the ECG?
    a. Bifascicular block
    b. Trifascicular block
    c. Atrial fibrillation with slow ventricular response
    d. Sinus bradycardia
    e. Complete heart block

DOI: 10.1201/9781003461456-15

2. Which of the following is NOT considered a common cause of the above ECG finding?

   a. Hypokalaemia

   b. Myocardial infarction

   c. Aortic stenosis

   d. Digoxin toxicity

   e. Beta-blockers

3. Which of the following rhythms would you be most likely to see if this patient went into cardiac arrest?

   a. Pulseless electrical activity (PEA)

   b. Ventricular fibrillation (VF)

   c. Pulseless VT (pVT)

   d. Asystole

   e. Torsade de pointes

☑ 1e Complete heart block

This ECG recording shows complete heart block evidenced by complete dissociation between P waves and broad complex QRS with independent atrial and ventricular rates. Looking closely there is likely left anterior fascicular block (LAFB) (left-axis deviation; small Q and tall R in I and aVL; small R and deep S in II, III and aVF; prolonged QRS) and right bundle branch block (RBBB). This is due to the ventricular escape rhythm arising from the region of either the left anterior or left posterior fascicle (distal to the site of block), producing QRS complexes with the appearance of RBBB plus either left posterior fascicular block (LPFB) or LAFB, respectively. The term trifascicular block would be suggested by bifascicular block with 1st or 2nd degree atrioventricular (AV) block, or fixed block of one fascicle (i.e. RBBB) with intermittent failure of the other two fascicles (i.e. alternating LAFB/LPFB). P waves are visible and QRS complexes are regular, which excludes atrial fibrillation.

☑ 2a Hypokalaemia

Hyperkalaemia rather than hypokalaemia may be associated with conduction abnormalities and bradycardia. ECG findings with severe hyperkalaemia (>7.0 mmol/L) include prolonged QRS interval with bizarre morphology, high-grade AV block with slow junctional and ventricular escape rhythms, other conduction blocks (bundle branch block or fascicular block), sinus bradycardia, slow atrial fibrillation (AF), sine wave appearance (pre-terminal event). All of the other options are possible causes for complete heart block, including right coronary artery or inferior myocardial infarction, and AV nodal blocking drugs (beta-blockers, calcium-channel blockers, digoxin). Other causes of AV block include inflammatory and autoimmune conditions such as rheumatic fever, myocarditis, systemic lupus erythematous, systemic sclerosis; infiltrative myocardial diseases such as amyloidosis, haemochromatosis, sarcoidosis; or following cardiac surgery, particularly surgery close to the septum, for example mitral valve repair. There is an idiopathic fibrous degenerative disorder of the conduction system referred to as Lenègre–Lev disease, which manifests as permanent complete AV block with cardiac pauses and syncopal episodes.

☑ 3d Asystole

Patients with complete heart block are at risk of asystolic arrest. Risk of asystole is increased in patients with Mobitz type II AV block, complete heart block with broad complex QRS, ventricular pause of >3 seconds or have had a recent asystole. It is extremely important to remember management of bradycardia, which includes an initial ABCDE assessment including monitoring of 3-lead ECG, BP and SpO$_2$ and a 12-lead ECG. If there is evidence of life-threatening signs, for example shock, syncope, myocardial ischaemia or heart failure, initial treatment is with an intravenous bolus of atropine

500 micrograms. This can be repeated to a maximum of 3 mg. If the response is unsatisfactory, alternatives include infusions of isoprenaline, adrenaline or dopamine. If pharmacological measures are unavailable or the response is unsatisfactory, be prepared to commence transcutaneous pacing; familiarise yourself with the pacing mode on the defibrillator. Note that glucagon can also be used in the context of suspected or confirmed beta-blocker or calcium-channel blocking drugs.

The cause of a cardiac arrest cannot be determined by the rhythm alone, but there are some associations. PEA is classically associated with either hypovolaemia or an outflow obstruction, for example massive PE. pVT and VF are seen more with electrolyte disturbances and myocardial infarction, particularly involving the pacemaker i.e. RCA territory. Torsades de pointes ('twisting of points') is a particular form of polymorphic VT associated with prolonged QT syndromes, which could be either congenital or associated with electrolyte disorders (low K^+, Mg^{2+}, Ca^{2+}) or caused by medications (for example, tricyclic antidepressants, haloperidol, loratadine, clarithromycin, ondansetron). The specific treatment along with generic resuscitation guidelines is to give 2 g magnesium IV and correct any other corresponding electrolyte abnormalities.

KEY LEARNING POINTS

- Complete heart block is typified by the dissociation of P waves and QRS complexes, which may often be broad and regular in this context.
- Complete heart block may be caused by a number of conditions including structural nodal issues, conductive system defects, electrolyte disturbances or toxidromes.
- Patients in complete heart block are at significant risk of an asystolic arrest and should be managed ideally in the resuscitation room with a defibrillator with pacing mode available.

Burning chest pain

A 31-year-old man with a background of relapse-remitting multiple sclerosis (MS) and ankylosing spondylitis presents with a 1 day history of left-sided chest pain radiating down his left arm associated with a new rash. The rash is described as burning and has a mild pruritic component. The patient tells you he has been advised by a pharmacist to use an antihistamine cream topically.

He denies pleuritic features of the chest pain, and states it is not crushing or pressing in nature and is not associated with dyspnoea, diaphoresis, nausea or vomiting, dizziness or radiation to the back.

Observations are within normal limits.

ECG is normal sinus rhythm.

The rash is shown below.

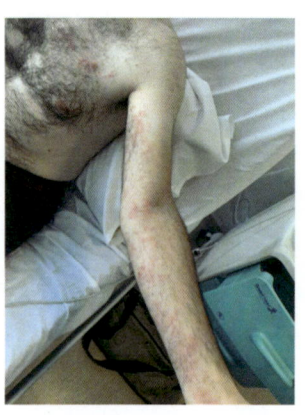 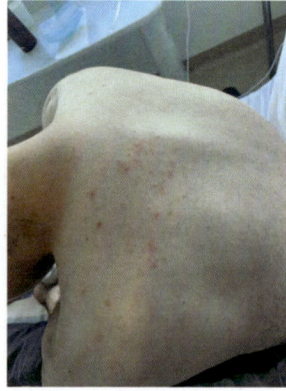 

1. Which of the following is the most likely diagnosis?

    a. Dermatitis herpetiformis

    b. Herpes simplex

    c. Impetigo

    d. Herpes zoster

    e. *Mycobacterium leprae*

DOI: 10.1201/9781003461456-16

2. If left untreated, which of the following could be a potential complication of the above presentation?

   a. Keratitis

   b. Retinitis

   c. Urinary retention

   d. Chronic pain

   e. All of the above

The patient's blood results come back showing normal renal function and liver function tests. The CRP is not raised, but you note the lymphocyte count is 0.67 and total WCC 4.71.

His medication history includes dimethyl fumarate (DMF), pregabalin, melatonin, sildenafil, solifenacin and tramadol.

He weighs approximately 70 kg.

3. What definitive treatment option would you consider given his current medications?

   a. Oral aciclovir 800 mg 5 times per day for 7 days

   b. Oral prednisolone 40 mg OD for 10–14 days with PPI cover

   c. Oral dapsone starting at 100 mg OD, titrated up to 300 mg for 7 days

   d. IV aciclovir 700 mg TDS for 5 days

   e. IV flucloxacillin 1 g QDS for 48 hours and then oral for a total of 10 days

☑ 1d Herpes zoster

This patient has the typical rash of shingles, which is caused by Herpes (Varicella) zoster. Herpes zoster usually begins with localised pain without visible skin change, often with associated systemic symptoms of headache, fever and malaise. After a few days, a red papular rash of fluid-filled vesicles is seen with new lesions erupting for several days. These papules either blister or become pustular before crusting over. Zoster can be differentiated from the other options as it is usually observed in a dermatomal distribution, T1 in this case. Dermatitis herpetiformis is an unusual condition associated with coeliac disease. The patient is typically 30–40 years old and presents with itchy blisters on the elbows, back, scalp and buttocks. Management is with a gluten free diet and dapsone. Impetigo is classically caused by *Staphylococcus* infection and presents with a painful rash resembling folliculitis with a 'golden' crust, often around the mouth and genital areas. It is extremely infectious and treated with either topical antibiotics (for example, fucidin) if localised or oral antibiotics (for example, flucloxacillin) if more widespread. Herpes simplex virus (HSV) presents in a similar way to shingles with papules and a raised vesicle filled with a clear fluid if uninfected. These infections are caused by two types of HSV, typically but not exclusively, with HSV-1 causing oral infections and HSV-2 causing genital infections.

☑ 2e All of the above

Herpes zoster infection can cause a variety of complications, the most common of which is post-herpetic neuralgia, which is chronic pain in the area affected by the zoster infection. However, there are a host of other rarer complications, such as transverse myelitis (which may cause urinary retention), Ramsay–Hunt syndrome (which may lead to keratitis or retinitis), superimposed bacterial infections, meningoencephalitis and visceral herpes zoster, which may present with severe abdominal pain. Post-herpetic neuralgia typically affects 1 in 5 people with shingles, though adults over 50 years old are at greater risk. Many will make a full recovery within a year, but symptoms last longer for some individuals, which can be quite debilitating. Non-medical management options include comfortable clothing, covering the area to avoid irritation and cold/ice packs. Medical management options include tricyclic antidepressants such as amitriptyline; medications used in chronic pain such as gabapentin, pregabalin or tramadol; or local treatments such as capsaicin cream or lidocaine patches.

☑ 3d IV aciclovir 700 mg TDS for 5 days

This patient has MS and is on DMF, an immunomodulatory therapy. It works by decreasing T cell counts (CD-8 more than CD-4) as well as shifting the state of B cells, myeloid cells and NK cells to a more anti-inflammatory state. The exact cellular mechanism of how DMF works is unclear. However, this puts him at risk of disseminated herpes zoster infection, which can lead to serious complications such as transverse myelitis and encephalitis. He should therefore be treated with high dose (10 mg/kg) IV aciclovir as an inpatient in the first instance, with referral to both infectious diseases and neurology teams. DMF should be stopped in disseminated infection but was continued in this case of localised shingles after neurology input. Oral aciclovir 800 mg 5 times per day for 7 days is the treatment for zoster in non-immunocompromised individuals, dapsone is used for the treatment of dermatitis herpetiformis, and flucloxacillin can be used in widespread impetigo.

KEY LEARNING POINTS

- Herpes zoster typically presents with a vesicular rash in a dermatomal distribution.
- Whilst long-term complications are rare in immunocompetent patients, careful safety net advice should be given, especially if discharging patients home.
- Medications that can depress the immune system may alter the best treatment for the patient. Ensure that you clarify all medications that a patient may be taking and seek specialist advice where appropriate.

CASE 17

Central chest pain

A 53-year-old man walks into the emergency department (ED) complaining of central chest pain behind the lower sternum with no radiation, 'sharp' in nature, 8/10 severity, not affected by position or inspiration and accompanied by profuse sweating last night. The pain subsides slightly after administration of paracetamol by the ED triage nurse.

His past medical history includes hypertension, hypercholesterolaemia and anxiety with infrequent panic attacks. He takes ramipril 5 mg and rosuvastatin 20 mg daily. He tells you his sister suffers with angina and his brother has diabetes. He has smoked 15 cigarettes per day for the last 30 years.

On examination, you note a raised BMI, warm peripheries but not clammy, normal vesicular breath sounds, normal heart sounds and no chest wall tenderness.

The initial ECG is shown below.

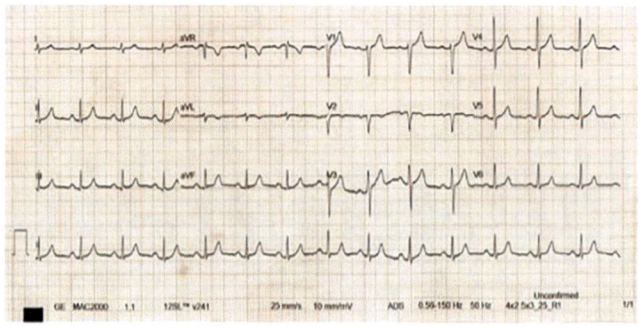

1. Which of the following is the best description of the ECG trace?

    a. Hyperacute T waves

    b. Normal ECG

    c. Posterior myocardial infarction

    d. Benign early repolarisation

    e. Wellens' syndrome

DOI: 10.1201/9781003461456-17

Whilst in the department, the patient reports that his chest pain has worsened; a repeat ECG is performed whilst he is experiencing the pain.

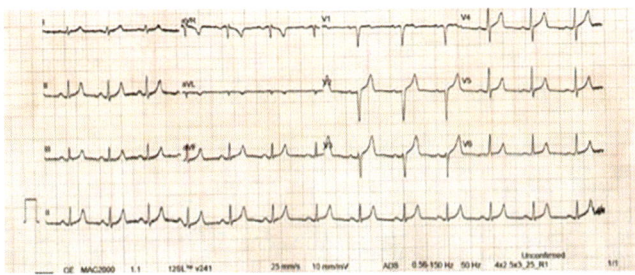 

2. Which of the following is the best description of the repeat ECG?

   a. Normal ECG

   b. Brugada syndrome

   c. Posterior myocardial infarction

   d. Hyperacute T waves and early ST elevation

   e. Non-specific T wave changes

On review of the bloods, the first Troponin T is 575 ng/L, and a repeat Troponin T 2 hours after is 966 ng/L.

The patient is pain free after sublingual glyceryl trinitrate (GTN) and intravenous morphine and has been commenced on treatment for acute coronary syndrome with aspirin, clopidogrel, fondaparinux and bisoprolol.

The cardiology team advise inpatient admission for further treatment and investigation. However, the patient would like to go home.

3. Which of the following is the best way to manage this situation?

   a. The patient is at high risk of ventricular arrhythmias and death, and therefore he cannot be allowed to leave hospital under any circumstance and must be held against his will

   b. Discuss with cardiology in an effort to expedite inpatient angiogram to be done today

   c. Call security, sign a Deprivation of Liberty Safeguards (DoLS) form and prevent him from leaving the department

   d. Administer lorazepam 4 mg and haloperidol 10 mg IM and move to observable cubicle

   e. Assess his capacity – if he has capacity, allow him to leave but arrange follow-up with the acute internal medicine ambulatory hot clinic tomorrow as a first point of contact and advise to dial for an ambulance if pain recurs

☑ 1a Hyperacute T waves

A feature of myocardial ischaemia which is not commonly seen but present here are broad, asymmetrically peaked or 'hyperacute' T waves. These are seen in the early stages of ST elevation myocardial infarction (STEMI) and often precede the appearance of ST elevation and subsequent Q waves. They are also seen with Prinzmetal angina, otherwise known as vasospastic angina, where the coronary arteries go into spasm caused by medications such as ephedrine and sumatriptan or recreational drugs including cocaine and amphetamines. The hyperacute T waves can be subtle, especially if there is no previous ECG available for comparison. Look again at the trace above and compare the size of the T wave to the QRS complex. Posterior myocardial infarction is suggested by changes in V1-V3 with horizontal ST depression, tall broad R waves and dominant R wave in V2. Posterior infarction is seen in 15–20% of STEMI but can also be seen in isolation. Benign early repolarisation ('high take-off' or 'J-point elevation') is commonly seen in young, healthy patients. There is often widespread concave ST elevation, predominantly in V2-5, notching at the J-point, and no reciprocal ST depression. Wellens' syndrome is characterised by biphasic or deeply inverted T waves in V2 and V3 with a history of recently resolved chest pain; it is highly specific for critical stenosis of the left anterior descending artery.

☑ 2d Hyperacute T waves and early ST elevation

The T waves in the anterior chest leads have become more peaked. V1 now shows pathological Q waves, which usually indicate current or previous myocardial infarction; Q waves are considered pathological if >40 ms (1 mm) wide, >2 mm deep, >25% of the depth of QRS complex. There is also very early ST elevation in the anterior chest leads compared to the first ECG, but it is not 2 mm, which would meet the criteria for STEMI thrombolysis. There are also subtle changes in leads II, III and aVF – note how the ST segment is starting to slope upwards. Brugada syndrome is a diagnosis based on ECG findings and clinical criteria. The 'Brugada sign' is a coved ST segment elevation >2 mm in more than one of leads V1-3 followed by a negative T wave. This must be accompanied by one of the following: ventricular fibrillation or polymorphic ventricular tachycardia, family history of sudden cardiac death under 45 years old, inducible ventricular tachycardia or nocturnal agonal respiration.

☑ 3e Assess his capacity – if he has capacity, allow him to leave but arrange follow-up with the acute internal medicine ambulatory hot clinic tomorrow as a first point of contact and advise to dial for an ambulance if pain recurs

The patient has had a significant myocardial infarction and is at risk of deterioration including the development of arrhythmias and death. He must be informed of these risks and if he has capacity to understand, retain, weigh up and communicate these, he cannot be held against his will in hospital. A common misconception is the need to sign a self-discharge form, but what you must do is clearly document your capacity assessment, as should any other witnessing clinicians or nursing staff. A reasonable option would be to offer a hot clinic follow-up appointment as this would provide an additional layer of safety rather than no follow-up at all. Direct access to cardiology is preferred but difficult to arrange in most healthcare settings.

KEY LEARNING POINTS

- Careful interpretation of the ECG can reveal early signs of acute coronary syndromes such as hyperacute T waves in the absence of other causes such as hyperkalaemia.
- Serial ECGs are useful for comparison as they will help to identify dynamic changes.
- Capacity assessments should be carefully documented in the patient's notes at the time of assessment with a full explanation of what was discussed including the risks of abstaining from acute treatment. However, this does not mean that follow-up appointments cannot be arranged as part of your safety net.

Chest pain and weakness

A 72-year-old woman presents following an episode of severe left-sided chest and back pain, radiating to the left side of the neck. This is associated with transient bilateral leg weakness. The patient was unable to walk for 1 hour but power to the lower limbs has slowly returned. The paramedic crew state at handover that she has no facial droop, arm or leg weakness or speech disturbance, but have brought her to the Hyper Acute Stroke Unit (HASU).

Past medical history includes hypertension, hypothyroidism and quiescent large vessel vasculitis (PET negative).

Initial observations are recorded as HR 83, BP 112/98, SpO_2 98% on room air, RR 14, afebrile, GCS 15/15. Current pain is reported as 4/10.

1. Which of the following investigations would NOT be included in your first investigation set?
   a. Non-contrast head CT
   b. ECG
   c. Chest radiograph
   d. Point-of-care ultrasound abdominal aorta and echo
   e. High sensitivity Troponin

DOI: 10.1201/9781003461456-18

The following imaging is performed.

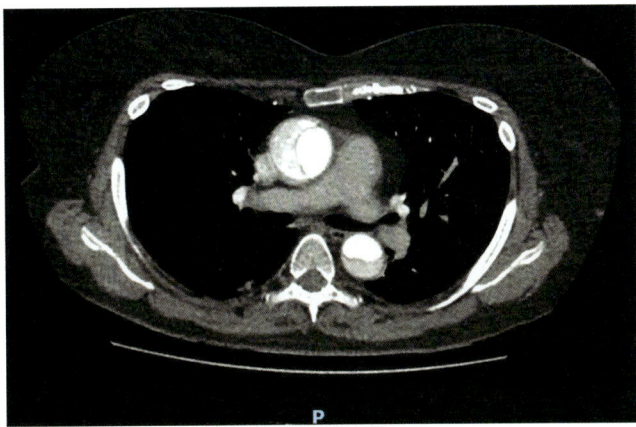

2. What is the diagnosis?

   a. Saddle pulmonary embolus

   b. Type B aortic dissection

   c. Dissection of infra-renal abdominal aorta

   d. Type A aortic dissection extending to the common iliac artery

   e. Malignant pericardial effusion

The patient remains stable in the department and repeat observations are unchanged.

3. Which of the following is the best definitive management option at this stage?

   a. Critical transfer to thoracic team for pericardial window and catheter placement

   b. Refer to local intensive care unit (ICU) for thrombolysis and right heart pressure management

   c. Referral to the vascular team for consideration of surgery

   d. Admit locally under the stroke team for anticoagulation and blood pressure control

   e. Critical transfer to cardiothoracic team for urgent surgery

☑ 1a Non-contrast CT

The differential is wide in this case but remember a ST elevation myocardial infarction (STEMI), especially inferior or posterior, could present with these symptoms and an ECG can quickly exclude this. Or there may be suggestions of a large PE (sinus tachycardia, right-axis deviation or the fabled S1Q3T3 pattern). Remember, lots of patients will have an ECG with the paramedic team – don't forget to review this and compare it to ones performed in the emergency department (ED) to assess for any evolving changes. A chest radiograph also has diagnostic value in this case to look for possible signs of aortic dissection. Key signs include a widened mediastinum, apical cap, depression of the left mainstem bronchus, obscuration of the aortic knob and pleural effusions. POCUS is an established part of modern EM. It can be rapidly used to visualise the abdominal aorta (to look for an aneurysm) and the heart (to look for general wall motion and pericardial effusions as well as signs of dissection). Specific protocols exist for unwell hypotensive patients (RUSH-ED and SHOCC scan), but do not delay definitive imaging such as CT if point-of-care scanning is not conclusive. Troponin could be elevated in a STEMI/NSTEMI, massive PE and extensive aortic dissection (especially Stanford A type involving the aortic root). At this stage, a non-contrast CT head would be least likely to provide information for a cause of the patient's symptoms. Although stroke or TIA would be on the differential list, the best modality for identifying the acute stroke in the ED would be a CT head and CT angiogram.

☑ 2d Type A aortic dissection extending to the common iliac artery

The aortagram shows a Stanford Type A aortic dissection extending from the aortic root to the right external iliac artery; there is also involvement of the right internal carotid (the end of the flap cannot be identified here). You can see the true lumen (bright white), which is slightly compressed by the crescentic shaped false lumen, which is darker grey due to delayed filling phase. This dissection is classified as a Stanford Type A due to the involvement of the ascending aorta (~60% of all dissections), whereas if only the descending aorta was involved this would be Stanford Type B. There is no aneurysmal component and no evidence of rupture on this scan. In this case, the renal arteries continue to be supplied from the true lumen as well as the mesenteric vessels, otherwise ischaemic bowel could complicate the clinical picture. The other commonly used classification system is the DeBakey classification, which has three types also grouped by anatomical features. The key risk factor for aortic dissection in this patient is the history of large vessel vasculitis. Other risk factors for aortic dissection include hypertension, atherosclerosis and connective tissue diseases.

☑ 3e Critical transfer to cardiothoracic team for urgent surgery

Type A aortic dissections carry a high mortality if left untreated due to involvement of the aortic root and valve as they have potential for myocardial ischaemia and cardiac arrest. Therefore, urgent referral and critical transfer (depending on local protocols) to the appropriate cardiothoracic team for surgical management should be arranged. Surgical techniques involve removing the ascending aorta, replacing it with a synthetic graft and the patient may also require aortic valve replacement. Uncomplicated Type B aortic dissections are often managed medically with blood pressure control alone. However, they may also require surgical management, particularly if any complications are present, such as rupture, renal/bowel/limb ischaemia or uncontrollable hypertension.

KEY LEARNING POINTS

- A careful, discriminatory approach should be given to initial investigations based on history, clinical examination and probable diagnoses.
- Aortic dissections have a typical crescenteric appearance on CT with the presence of a true lumen and a false lumen.
- Stanford Type A dissections should be referred urgently to the local cardiothoracic team for surgical management due to involvement of the aortic root and high mortality.

Chest pain in an intravenous drug user

A 35-year-old man with a background of intravenous drug use is bought to the emergency department with profuse diarrhoea and also complains of severe central pleuritic chest pain. He admits to taking over-the-counter laxatives and reports he last injected crack cocaine 4 days ago. He informs you he has a history of infective endocarditis (around 10 years ago) and spent a number of weeks in hospital.

Initial observations are recorded as HR 110, BP 105/60, SpO$_2$ 95% on room air, RR 24, temperature 39°C (102.2°F). He looks pale, clammy and generally unwell.

Examination of the chest reveals coarse crepitations in the right base and the abdomen is generally tender although not peritonitic.

A venous blood gas (VBG) reveals pH 7.465, BE +4.2, HCO$_3^-$ 26.9, Lactate 0.8, Hb 81.

A chest radiograph is performed.

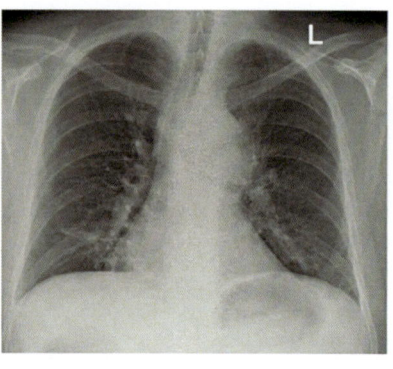

1. What is the single best description of the chest radiograph?

    a. Right basal atelectasis and bilateral hilar enlargement

    b. Right lower lobe consolidation

    c. Widened mediastinum and right basal linear atelectasis

    d. No abnormality detected

    e. Mediastinal free air and surgical emphysema

DOI: 10.1201/9781003461456-19

You review the laboratory blood results and note the following: Hb 76, MCV 64.9, WCC 9.47, CRP 185, Na⁺ 125, K⁺ 4.3, creatinine 91, D-dimer 3150.

On the basis of the above results, a CT pulmonary angiogram is organised.

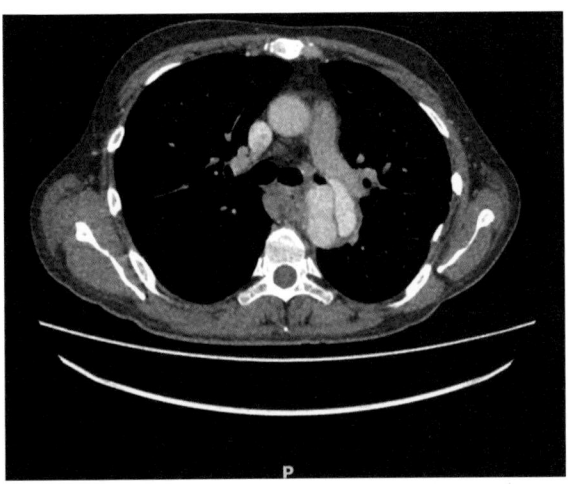

2. What is the most significant finding on the CT which may explain the patient's presentation?

   a. Peripheral emboli with abscess formation suggestive of infective emboli

   b. Bilateral basal consolidation and right sided pleural effusion

   c. Soft tissue mass in the mediastinum suggestive of lymphoma

   d. Large saddle embolus with evidence of right heart strain

   e. Extravasation of contrast from the anterior aspect of the descending aorta

3. What is the most appropriate management based on the above findings?

   a. Flucloxacillin 2 g IV, refer to infectious diseases team for further investigation

   b. Group & save, blood cultures, cefuroxime 1.5 g IV + 480 mg gentamicin IV, refer to cardiothoracic team and infectious diseases team

   c. Treatment dose low molecular weight heparin, co-amoxiclav 1.2 g IV, refer to acute internal medicine team

   d. Co-amoxiclav 1.2 g IV, refer to haematology team for inpatient biopsy of mediastinal mass

   e. Insertion of arterial line, refer to intensive care unit, contact interventional radiology to consider catheter-directed thrombolysis

☑ 1c Widened mediastinum and right basal linear atelectasis

The history of pleuritic chest pain with a temperature and borderline oxygen saturations should raise high index of suspicion for a pneumonia and there is possible evidence of right lower consolidation. However, this may be atelectasis. More importantly, there is increased left hilar shadowing and loss of clear aortic knuckle. This is the first evidence in this case that there may be evidence of aortic pathology. When considering aortic dissection, a number of radiographic signs on a plain chest radiograph can be found including a widened mediastinum >8–8.8 cm at level of aortic notch, double/irregular aortic contour and inward displacement of atherosclerotic calcification. However, it is important to remember that assessing the mediastinum width can be complicated by magnification that can occur in anterior-posterior chest radiographs. Furthermore, the presence of periaortic or mediastinal haematoma can cause signs of obscuring the aortic notch, deviation of mediastinal structures, increased thickness of left and/or right paratracheal stripe, apical capping.

☑ 2e Extravasation of contrast from the anterior aspect of the descending aorta

Due to this patient's background of intravenous drug use and previous infective endocarditis, he is at significantly increased risk of septic emboli so a low index of suspicion for cross-sectional imaging is required. There are several findings of note on this CT; there are bilateral small pleural effusions with patchy consolidation suggestive of atelectasis, and also a significantly enlarged spleen. However, the most concerning finding is an extravasation of contrast from the anterior aspect of the descending thoracic aorta (seen 00m10s). The patient is septic, and therefore a mycotic thoracic aneurysm was the most likely culprit. The Hb of 76, the severe nature of his pain and the CT findings indicated that there was indeed ongoing leakage from the aneurysm. Mycotic aneurysms are a small minority of aortic aneurysms and common risk factors include intravenous drug use, infective endocarditis, immunosuppression, atherosclerotic plaque or prosthetic devices (stents and grafts). The vessel wall becomes infected by bacteria and a false aneurysm forms, which is extremely prone to rupture with associated haemorrhage. The most commonly involved organisms are *Staphylococcus aureus* and *Salmonella* spp.

☑ 3b Group & save, blood cultures, cefuroxime 1.5 g IV + 480 mg gentamicin IV, refer to cardiothoracic team and infectious diseases team

Though this patient will require specialist input from multiple specialty teams, it is most important to urgently refer to the cardiothoracic team in order to treat the leaking aneurysm before further complications arise. Depending on local service availability where you are working, you may also need to refer to the vascular team. According to sepsis protocols, he will require prompt administration of broad-spectrum intravenous anti-biotics as per local microbiology guidelines. It is best practice to send off blood cultures prior to the administration of antibiotics as this is the best chance to isolate the causative organism. It may be prudent to discuss this complex case directly with the microbiology team to ensure adequate antimicrobial cover is provided. He is also anaemic and requires group & save in case of further bleeding requiring blood transfusion. If he had been hypertensive, he would also have required blood pressure control; most commonly used is intravenous labetalol, which can be given in boluses or infusion and should be used alongside invasive blood pressure monitoring with an arterial line. His hyponatraemia will also need careful investigation and treatment. Remember non-judicious administration of IV fluids may cause it to fall further and over-rapid correction runs the risk of central pontine myelinolysis.

KEY LEARNING POINTS

- There are a number of radiological signs associated with aortic dissection that can be found on a plain chest radiograph, including a widened mediastinum.
- Remember that host risk factors and lifestyle are important when considering causes of acute aortic dissection.
- Multidisciplinary team input is important in complex cases, particularly where infection may complicate the presentation.

Complex headache

A 50-year-old man presents to the emergency department (ED) complaining of progressively worsening headaches one month after undergoing revision right tympanoplasty for recurrent cholesteatoma. He has attended different EDs on multiple occasions during this time. He was seen by the ENT team a week before this presentation, who discharged him with oral antibiotics. The pain is described as a severe, 'squeezing' sensation in the right occiput radiating around to his temple and is worse on movement or speech. He has had no discharge from the ear, no fever or neurological symptoms.

Initial observations are recorded as HR 100, BP 130/74, SpO_2 100% on room air, RR 17, temperature 36.8°C (98.2°F).

On examination, you note some tenderness around the post-auricular incision site, but the pinna and mastoid appear normal.

He is referred to ENT and a CT head scan is arranged.

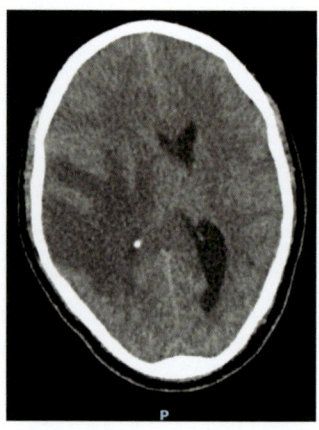 

1. What is the single best description of the CT findings?

   a. Intraparenchymal haemorrhage within the temporal lobe

   b. Left temporal lobe abscess with no signs of mass effect

   c. Right occipital lobe abscess with signs of mass effect

   d. Right temporal lobe abscess with signs of mass effect

   e. Uncomplicated left-sided cholesteatoma

DOI: 10.1201/9781003461456-20

The case is discussed with the local neurosurgeons who accept the case for urgent neurosurgical drainage.

2. Which of the following is also recommended in all patients with brain abscesses?

   a. Corticosteroids

   b. Anticonvulsant prophylaxis

   c. Analgesia

   d. IV antibiotics prior to surgery

   e. Antiemetic

He is transferred to a local neurosurgical unit for an emergency craniotomy and excision of brain abscess.

Culture of specimens collected during the operation grows *Staphylococcus aureus*. He remains intubated for several weeks as there are complications to his recovery, and he is treated with a complex high-dose antibiotic regimen.

When extubated he is found to have a visual deficit in all fields. The aetiology of his visual impairment may be multifactorial.

3. Which one of these antibiotics is associated with visual loss?

   a. Tazocin

   b. Linezolid

   c. Meropenem

   d. Ceftriaxone

   e. Flucloxacillin

☑ 1d Right temporal lobe abscess with signs of mass effect

There is a hypoattenuating lesion in the right temporal lobe with surrounding area of oedema, suggestive of intracranial abscess formation. The slightly hyperattenuating regions may represent blood, but the primary finding is of the right temporal lobe abscess. Effacement of the lateral ventricle, midline shift and early uncal herniation are present, which are all signs of mass effect. If intravenous contrast was given, you would also expect to see peripheral enhancement of the low-density lesion. MRI is more sensitive than CT and diffusion-weighted sequences can help to distinguish abscesses from other ring enhancing lesions by evidence of diffusion restriction within the abscess cavity. A cholesteatoma is histologically equivalent to an epidermoid cyst and is composed of desquamated keratinizing stratified squamous epithelium that forms a mass. Patients may present with otorrhoea, conductive hearing loss or dizziness or be asymptomatic. They are best evaluated using MRI, but on CT you may see a non-dependent, homogenous soft tissue mass with a focal area of bone destruction.

☑ 2b Anticonvulsant prophylaxis

A tricky one here, but the key feature is that this will be urgent surgery and so in the case where a patient is taken straight to theatre, it is recommended that antibiotics are held until a sample can be taken intraoperatively for culture. Otherwise, empirical antibiotics are the first-line treatment and should be given according to the local microbiology policy; note that the consideration of antibiotic choice will include its permeability across the blood–brain barrier. All patients with brain abscess should be given anticonvulsant prophylaxis with first-line agents, for example, levetiracetam, sodium valproate or carbamazepine. The use of corticosteroids is controversial. They can be a life-saving treatment when a patient is acutely decompensating as they quickly reduce the oedema. However, practice differs between clinicians; some argue that dexamethasone improves antibiotic treatment through reduction of the oedema, whereas others think that immunosuppression has a negative impact on outcomes. A recent systematic review and meta-analysis published found no increased mortality with use of dexamethasone.

☑ 3b Linezolid

Linezolid is an oxazolidinone antibiotic whose uses include methicillin-resistant *Staphylococcus aureus* (MRSA), vancomycin-resistant enterococci (VRE) and drug-resistant tuberculosis. Visual deficits secondary to linezolid-induced optic neuropathy typically develop after prolonged use, with the majority of cases improving following the cessation of linezolid although some cases have residual deficits. It has been suggested that patients receiving treatment for 28 days or longer should be followed up to assist early identification of optic neuropathy and early withdrawal of linezolid. Oxazolidinones inhibit bacterial protein synthesis by binding to the 70S ribosome. It is hypothesised that the aetiology of the toxicity is related to mitochondrial dysfunction, as their function is known to be more susceptible to disruption in retinal ganglion cells. Isoniazid, ethambutol and fluoroquinolone antibiotics are other antibiotics that are associated with optic-neuropathy, as well as exposure to ethylene glycol, methanol, and deficiency of vitamin B12, folate and thiamine.

KEY LEARNING POINTS

- Have a low threshold for imaging post-operative patients representing to the ED on several occasions and seek a specialist opinion.
- Antibiotics can be held until operative intervention and biopsy if a patient is clinically stable and there are no signs of meningitis, as this will increase positive yields.
- Linezolid is associated with retinal toxicity, especially in high doses or prolonged courses.

Complication of alcohol excess

A 35-year-old man is transferred to the emergency department from a nearby hospital. He tells you that he had three seizures and after that suffered severe tearing chest and upper abdominal pain. He denies vomiting or haematemesis. Bowels last opened yesterday. He has significant alcohol intake of approximately 1 L of vodka per day.

Initial observations are recorded as HR 125, BP 135/86, SpO$_2$ 98% on 4 L via nasal cannula, RR 30, temperature 37.2°C (98.9°F), GCS 15/15. On inspection, the patient is sitting up, profusely sweating and looks restless. He does not tolerate lying flat. In a semi-recumbent position, the abdomen is diffusely tender, and you note reduced air entry on both lower zones of the chest.

A 12-lead ECG is performed, which shows sinus tachycardia.

An arterial blood gas (ABG) is taken as part of his initial work-up.

ⓘ POCT ARTERIAL BLOOD GAS

Status: **Final result**

Component Ref Range & Units	1mo ago		
Source	**Arterial**		
pH	7.456^	**Deoxyhaemoglobin** %	2.4
Comment: Value above reference range		**Oxyhaemoglobin** %	95.3
Carbon Dioxide Partial Pressure kPa	6.05^	**Saturated Oxygen** %	97.5
Comment: Value above reference range		**Carboxyhaemoglobin** %	1.6
Oxygen Partial Pressure kPa	11.1	**Methaemoglobin** %	0.7
Potassium mmol/L	3.6	**Bilirubin** micromol/l	0ˇ
Sodium mmol/L	145	Comment: Value below reference range	
Ionised Calcium mmol/L	1.02ˇ	**Standard Base Excess** mmol/L	8.1^
Comment: Value below reference range		Comment: Value above reference range	
Chloride mmol/L	104	**Standard Bicarbonate** mmol/L	30.8^
Glucose mmol/L	6.5^	Comment: Value above reference range	
Comment: Value above reference range		**Haematocrit** %	40.5
Lactate mmol/L	1.6	**Oxygen Tension at 50% Saturation** kPa	3.32
Urea mmol/L	3.2	**Oxygen Content** mmol/L	7.9
Creatinine micromol/l	83.3		
Total Haemoglobin g/l	132	Oxi compensated for HbF	

DOI: 10.1201/9781003461456-21

1. What condition would you NOT include in your differential diagnosis based on the clinical history and available investigations?

    a. Pancreatitis

    b. Boerhaave syndrome

    c. Aortic dissection

    d. Acute appendicitis

    e. Diabetic ketoacidosis

You review the CT performed at the referring hospital.

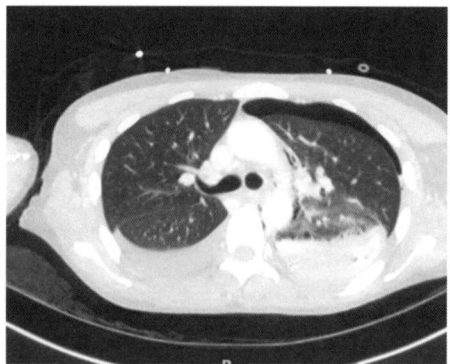 

2. Which of the following is the best description of the abnormal findings?

    a. There is pneumomediastinum and a left-sided pneumothorax with bibasal effusions. There is a left-sided intercostal drain with the tip pointed posteriorly and upwards

    b. There is evidence of multiple posterior left-sided rib fractures and associated left-sided pneumothorax. There is no splenic injury in the imaged portion of the upper abdomen. Secondary survey is advised to check for further injury

    c. There is evidence of left-sided bronchiectasis with a large basal effusion. Does this patient have a significant history of smoking?

    d. There are bilateral pleural effusions noted. Note is made of a left-sided intercostal drain with the tip appearing to abut against the thoracic aorta

    e. There is evidence of a thoracic aortic aneurysm rupture with moderation volume left-sided haemothorax. Urgent surgical chest drain placement is advised, with discussion with cardiothoracic surgeons

The patient is referred to the general surgeons and intensive care unit.

You discuss the case with the attending general surgical registrar, and he mentions Mackler's triad.

3. Which of the following describes Mackler's triad?

    a. Vomiting, epigastric pain, dyspnoea

    b. Vomiting, lower chest pain, surgical emphysema

    c. Vomiting, elevated JVP, muffled heart sounds

    d. Hypotension, elevated JVP, muffled heart sounds

    e. Hypotension, lower chest pain, surgical emphysema

☑ 1e Diabetic ketoacidosis

The potential cause of this man's symptoms is wide, and the history is relatively limited. With the information provided, the top differential diagnoses to identify or exclude would be pancreatitis (suggested by the history of alcohol excess and the upper abdominal pain), aortic dissection (suggested by the diaphoresis, tearing chest pain and sudden onset), and oesophageal rupture or Boerhaave syndrome (suggested by tearing chest and abdominal pain, clinical signs of pleural effusion and the inability to lie flat). Though atypical for acute appendicitis, the suggestion of sepsis along with a tender abdomen could indicate a perforated appendix and peritonitis. Diabetic ketoacidosis is essentially excluded by the ABG results showing normoglycaemia, and absence of metabolic acidosis. It is important to thoroughly assess any patients who are transferred from other hospitals to your department, even if they are expected by a specialist inpatient team, and particularly if they are unwell. Review the clinical history, examine the patient, review any investigations that have already been performed and arrange further investigations as indicated.

☑ 2a There is pneumomediastinum and a left-sided pneumothorax with bibasal effusions. There is a left-sided intercostal drain with the tip pointed posteriorly and upwards

In the lung windowed CT image provided, the striking abnormalities are a moderate volume left-sided pneumothorax with bilateral pleural effusions. There is also a left-sided surgical chest drain with the tip pointed posteriorly and to the apex. The tip is compressed against the lung parenchyma (see 00m11s), which might account for the incomplete drainage of air. There is also pneumomediastinum (see 00m16s), all suggestive of a radiological diagnosis of Boerhaave syndrome or oesophageal rupture. There are no rib fractures, making a traumatic pneumothorax less likely, and the thoracic and upper abdominal aorta appears to be of a normal diameter excluding aortic aneurysm. In suspected Boerhaave syndrome, administration of oral contrast alongside intravenous contrast for the CT can help identify the site of leak. Rupture of the oesophagus occurs due to forceful ejection of the gastric contents against a closed upper oesophageal sphincter. The most common location of rupture is the left posterolateral part of the thoracic oesophagus around 3–6 cm above the oesophageal hiatus (seen in this cine loop).

☑ 3b Vomiting, lower chest pain, surgical emphysema

Mackler's triad consists of vomiting, chest pain and surgical emphysema. Other symptoms of Boerhaave syndrome are epigastric and back pain, dyspnoea and shock. Despite being a logical sequence of events (vomiting leading to chest pain and then the surgical emphysema), it is said to be present in only 14% of patients. Hypotension, elevated JVP and muffled heart sounds are Beck's triad seen with pericardial effusion/

tamponade. Oesophageal rupture can include mediastinitis, oesophagopleural fistula, pneumonia and empyema. Mediastinitis and sepsis can be fatal but this is dramatically reduced when the condition is identified and treated early. Surgical intervention is usually required, but there is emerging use of alternative methods such as oesophageal stenting. Even with treatment, the mortality rate can reach up to 35% and so this must be treated as a surgical emergency.

KEY LEARNING POINTS

- Don't forget to review the blood glucose as hyperglycaemia can be a medical mimic of a surgical abdomen – normal in this case on the blood gas.
- CT with oral and intravenous contrast is helpful in Boerhaave syndrome as it can help identify the source of the oesophageal perforation.
- Patients should be resuscitated appropriately with early ICU input as mortality rates can be as high as 35%.

Complication of HIV

A 48-year-old Romanian man presents with a 3-week history of worsening abdominal pain. He states he has not opened his bowels properly for 2 weeks, only passing small amounts of hard stool every couple of days. He was seen twice in his local hospital and both times discharged with normal blood test results, but no further investigations. His pain has significantly worsened today, and he has vomited three times. He was diagnosed with HIV a month prior to presentation and has been started on anti-retroviral medications. His other past medical history includes syphilis, genital warts, anaemia, previous perforated peptic ulcer and a history of inguinal hernia repair.

Initial observations are recorded as HR 91, BP 119/76, SpO$_2$ 98% on room air, RR 17, temperature 36.7°C (98.1°F). On examination, the abdomen is mildly distended with marked epigastric tenderness and localised guarding.

A venous blood gas (VBG) is performed, which reveals pH 7.47, pO$_2$ 11.7, pCO$_2$ 4.2, Lactate 3.2, Urea 7, Creatinine 89, Hb 109.

A CT abdomen & pelvis with contrast is arranged.

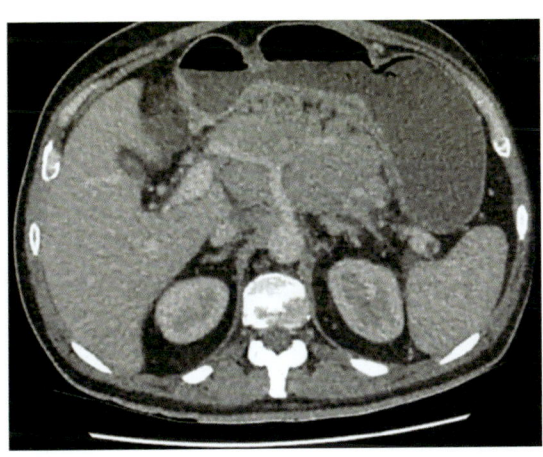

DOI: 10.1201/9781003461456-22

1.   What is the most noticeable abnormality?
     a.   Duodenal perforation with evident free gas in the upper abdomen
     b.   Adhesional small bowel obstruction with upstream dilatation of the stomach
     c.   Pancreatic adenocarcinoma causing gastric outlet obstruction
     d.   Extrinsic compression of proximal duodenum and mesenteric vessels
     e.   Faecal impaction with no obvious dilation of small or large bowel

Bloods are taken including FBC, U&E, LFTs, bone profile, coagulation profile and group & screen.

2.   Which of the following describes the best next management steps?
     a.   Insert NG tube, IV crystalloid fluid, antiemetic and analgesia; refer to infectious diseases and general surgeons
     b.   Ensure kept NBM, IV crystalloid fluid, antiemetic and analgesia; refer to general surgeons for urgent laparotomy
     c.   Draw additional blood for haemoglobinopathy screen, lactate dehydrogenase (LDH) and reticulocyte count; refer to haematology
     d.   Administer broad-spectrum IV antibiotics and IV crystalloid fluid; refer to hepato-biliary medicine
     e.   Insert NG tube, IV crystalloid fluid, antiemetic & analgesia; refer to vascular surgery

The patient continues to deteriorate rapidly during his admission.

A lymphocyte subset count is performed and presented below.

Lymphocyte Subsets (CD4)

Component	
Ref Range & Units	1mo ago
CD3 Percentage	80.3
57–87 %	
CD3 Absolute	1.97
0.87–2.51 x 10⁹/L	
CD4 Percentage	9.30ᵥ
31–61 %	
CD4 Absolute	0.23ᵥ
0.44–.47 x 10⁹/L	
CD4/CD3 Percentage	9.3ᵥ
31–61 %	
CD4/CD3 Absolute	0.229ᵥ
0.56–1.46 x 10⁹/L	
CD8/CD3 Percentage	62.4ᵃ
10–36 %	
CD8/CD3 Absolute	1.53ᵃ
0.25–0.99 x 10⁹/L	
CD4:CD8 Ratio	0.15ᵥ
0.54–2.97	

3. Which diagnoses could account for the findings on the CT abdomen & pelvis imaging based on these laboratory results?

   a. *Pneumocystis jiroveci*

   b. Visceral leishmaniasis

   c. *Toxoplasmosis gondii*

   d. Cryptosporidiosis

   e. Burkitt's lymphoma

☑ 1d Extrinsic compression of proximal duodenum and mesenteric vessels

The CT abdomen & pelvis shows an extremely large homogenous para-aortic mass, suggestive of para-aortic lymphadenopathy with associated compression of the duodenum and gross dilatation of the stomach due to gastric outflow obstruction. The mass is separate to the pancreas, with the pancreas appearing to lie anterior to it. Although there is duodenal obstruction, there are no dilated small bowel loops or fluid level within the more distal small bowel suggestive of small bowel obstruction, which can commonly be caused by adhesions. Additionally, there is no free fluid or gas suggestive of perforation. Compression of the mesenteric vessels leads to ischaemia of the bowel. In ischaemic bowel, the imaging findings can vary, but a number of features are common in advanced acute cases: increased bowel wall thickness, pneumatosis intestinalis (gas in bowel wall), pneumotosis portalis (gas in portal vein or mesenteric vein) and pneumoperitoneum.

☑ 2a Insert NG tube, IV crystalloid fluid, antiemetic and analgesia; refer to infectious diseases and general surgeons

It is appropriate to place a nasogastric tube in order to decompress the very distended stomach, provide IV fluid replacement as well as adequate analgesia and antiemetics for symptomatic relief. This patient certainly needs to be reviewed by the general surgical team to determine if operative intervention is required, but the infectious diseases team must also be involved early on in order to help guide further investigation to determine the cause of the lymphadenopathy in a patient with newly diagnosed HIV. Further investigations such as CD4 count, viral load, LDH and EBV and CMV serology should also be considered in this patient. However, these are usually requested by the specialist team rather than during the emergency department work-up. If time allows, the case will need to be discussed in a multidisciplinary team meeting with the general surgeons, infectious diseases and radiologists to consider best next management (for example, stenting, laparotomy, CT-guided biopsy and further imaging for staging).

☑ 3e Burkitt's lymphoma

High HIV viral load and low CD4 count can increase risk for developing non-Hodgkin's lymphomas such as Burkitt's lymphoma or other neoplasms such as Kaposi's sarcoma and also opportunistic infections. Burkitt's lymphoma may present with constitutional symptoms such as drenching sweating, unexplained fever, anorexia and weight loss as well as classical lymphadenopathy. In Western settings, Burkitt's may present with an abdominal mass or symptoms of bowel obstruction. Prompt diagnosis is necessary by biopsy, as it is quite aggressive. Gastrointestinal Kaposi's sarcoma is not uncommon; it is usually asymptomatic but may present with GI bleeding due to the angio-proliferative nature of the lesions and is best visualised via endoscopy. Toxoplasmosis may cause lymphadenopathy but this is normally peripheral and in a cervical distribution making it unlikely in this case. There is no shortness of breath or cough, which is commonly seen with *Pneumocystis*, and no diarrhoeal symptoms associated with Cryptosporidiosis, making these also unlikely diagnoses. Visceral leishmaniasis is characterised by symptoms of weight loss, fever, anaemia and hepatosplenomegaly rather than lymphadenopathy. Most cases are seen in Brazil, East Africa and India.

KEY LEARNING POINTS

- Axial imaging such as CT scanning should be performed in unexplained severe abdominal pain over abdominal radiography in the acute setting as the diagnostic yield is much higher.
- Wide bore nasogastric tube placement and replacement of fluids and electrolytes should be promptly constituted in acute bowel obstruction.
- Consider unusual causes of bowel obstruction in association with newly diagnosed or poorly controlled HIV such as lymphoma, sarcoma and opportunistic infections.
- Burkitt's lymphoma is very treatable if picked up early and can have a good prognosis with treatment.

CASE 23

Dazed and confused

A 58-year-old Indian man attended the emergency department (ED) after arriving back to the UK from a trip to Kenya. He tells you he first went to a hospital there after having seizure-like activity. He was diagnosed with an ischaemic stroke and discharged. Over the following month, his family reported a behavioural change, low mood, reduced mobility and confusion. He re-presented to the hospital in Kenya with a fever after falling at home, but tells you investigations were negative, including lumbar puncture. The family inform you that his brother had glioblastoma and his father had Parkinson's disease.

Initial observations are recorded as HR 65, BP 113/79, SpO_2 98% on room air, RR 16, temperature 37.1°C (98.8°F), GCS 13/15 (E3 V4 M6). The patient appears drowsy and confused. Clinical examination is otherwise normal with no focal neurological findings.

1. Which of the following would you request as your initial investigations?
   a. FBC/U&E/CRP, chest radiograph, CT head non-contrast
   b. FBC/U&E/CRP/LFT, malaria screen, blood cultures
   c. FBC/U&E/CRP/LFT, malaria screen, blood cultures, urine dip, CT intracranial angiogram
   d. FBC/U&E/CRP/LFT, malaria screen, blood cultures, chest radiograph, urine dip, CT head non-contrast
   e. FBC/U&E/CRP/LFT, blood cultures, chest radiograph, urine dip

The patient presents a CD containing MRI images from the hospital in Kenya, which are uploaded to the imaging system.

DOI: 10.1201/9781003461456-23

You look at the T2 FLAIR axial images and note the following appearances.

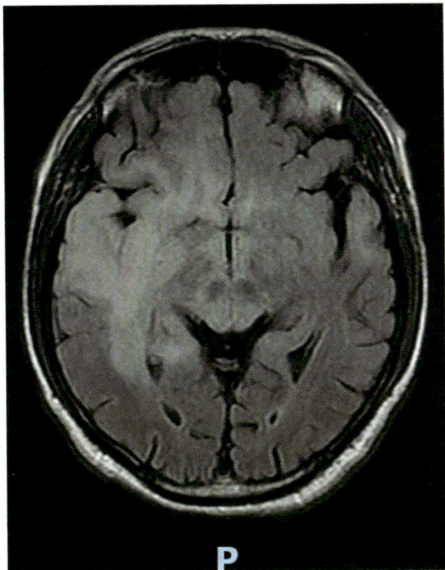

2. Which of the following would you NOT include in your list of differential diagnoses based on this imaging?
   a. HIV encephalitis
   b. Progressive multifocal leukoencephalopathy
   c. Primary central nervous system (CNS) lymphoma
   d. Herpes simplex encephalitis
   e. Virchow–Robin spaces (perivascular spaces)

3. Which symptoms are most in keeping with a temporo-parietal lesion?
   a. Motor deficit with behavioural change
   b. Hemianopia with macular sparing or problems with visual recognition
   c. Sensory disturbance, memory problems and emotional change
   d. Confusion, nausea and headache
   e. Dysphasia and dyslexia

☑ 1d FBC/U&E/CRP/LFT, malaria screen, blood cultures, chest radiograph, urine dip, CT head non-contrast

In summary, we have a man who has had a fever, recently travelled to a tropical country, and during travel has sustained a neurological insult. He now presents with drowsiness and confusion, suggesting ongoing involvement of the cerebrum in an underlying disease process. Based on the limited history and examination, differential diagnoses could include bacterial infection, viral encephalitis, cerebral malaria, HIV, autoimmune disorders and malignancy. Therefore, baseline bloods for inflammatory markers, renal and liver function are needed alongside blood cultures, malaria screen, chest radiograph and urine sample for dipstick testing and culture. HIV testing would also be advisable at this stage. Following more thorough assessment, it is likely that he will require further investigation, including neuroimaging. A CT head non-contrast could be considered in the ED especially if more advanced imaging such as MRI will be delayed. The primary pathologies it may reveal are large bleeds, mass effect, hydrocephalus and brain abscess although a contrast enhanced scan would be more useful in this context. CT intracranial angiogram would be indicated if acute ischaemic stroke was suggested.

☑ 2e Virchow–Robin spaces (perivascular spaces)

The MRI slice shows a large area of white matter hyperintensity (WMH) in the temporo-parietal lobes. White matter is the deeper part of the brain, consisting of glial cells and myelinated axons that connect the various grey matter areas. The differential list for this is wide including hypoxic/ischaemic (atherosclerosis, CADASIL, amyloid angiopathy), inflammatory (multiple sclerosis, systemic lupus erythematosus [SLE], sarcoidosis), infectious (HIV, progressive multifocal leukoencephalopathy), toxic/metabolic (B12 deficiency, carbon monoxide poisoning, central pontine myelinolysis) and trauma (radiotherapy, post-contusion). There can also be normal causes of WMH, such as Virchow–Robin spaces, but these follow cerebrospinal fluid (CSF) on all sequences and are not associated with neurological symptoms or signs. This is the 'odd one out' in this question. When narrowing down the potential pathological causes, it is important to consider patient age, geographical location, travel history and presenting symptoms, as well as the patterns of white matter disease. In this case of a returning traveller, one should appreciate that infective processes present more commonly and so herpes simplex or HIV encephalitis should be considered strongly until excluded. Tuberculosis is also a possibility, and in these cases, MRI might show a rounded tuberculoma with surrounding parenchymal change or TB meningeal changes. T2 FLAIR sequences suppress bright white CSF and is useful for looking for brain parenchymal changes.

☑ 3c Sensory disturbance, memory problems and emotional change

The somatosensory gyrus is in the parietal lobe and lesions here can lead to sensory disturbances and hemispatial neglect. The temporal lobe is involved in long-term memory, decision-making and emotional response. Frontal lesions have a diverse range of presentations, but commonly present with behavioural and personality changes, and inability to problem-solve. Hemianopia with macular sparing or problems with visual recognition would suggest an occipital lobe pathology. Remember a temporo-parietal lesion may present with visual changes if the optic radiation is affected too. Confusion, nausea and headache are more general symptoms of raised intracranial pressure and cerebral inflammation and not specific to temporo-parietal lesions. And lastly, dysphasia and dyslexia are most likely to be present in a dominant hemisphere parietal lesion.

KEY LEARNING POINTS

- Think widely about investigations in complex cases, particularly in those arriving from another centre or abroad. Each test must be rationalised for its diagnostic value in the clinical context.
- White matter hyperintensities are brain lesions that hyperintense on FLAIR MRI images. Causes can be wide ranging, from dementia, nutritional deficiencies and toxins, to infections and stroke.
- Temporo-parietal lesions typically present as sensory disturbance, memory problems and emotional change.

CASE 24

Do you think it's from the vaccine?

A 66-year-old Asian man presents to the emergency department complaining of 3 months of dry cough and shortness of breath on exertion. He reports that he first noticed the cough 10 days following his first COVID vaccination (Pfizer/BioNTech, mRNA). He denies fever, chest pain, dizziness or collapse. He feels the cough worsened after the second dose of the vaccine, and he also noticed swelling of the lower legs and face. He has a ten pack per year smoking history but no other past medical history.

Initial observations are recorded as HR 130, BP 150/90, SpO$_2$ 94% on room air, RR 32, temperature 36.8°C (98.6°F). There is reduced air entry bibasally with transmitted upper airway sounds. JVP is not visible, there are quiet heart sounds with a moderate pansystolic murmur and mild pedal oedema. You observe desaturation to 84% on movement during examination.

ECG shows sinus tachycardia with frequent ventricular ectopics. FBC, U&E, coagulation profile with fibrinogen and Troponin T are sent.

Wells score is calculated as 4.5 and a CTPA is performed.

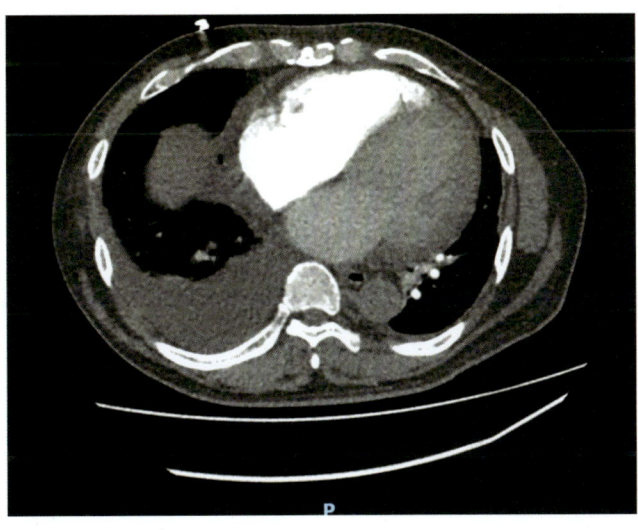

DOI: 10.1201/9781003461456-24

1. Which of the following best describes the observed abnormalities?

   a. No large pulmonary embolism, dilated left ventricle, large pericardial effusion and impending tamponade

   b. No large pulmonary embolism, dilated left ventricle, pericardial effusion, bilateral pleural effusions, dilated hepatic veins

   c. No large pulmonary embolism, dilated left ventricle, small pericardial effusion, bilateral pleural effusions, reflux of contrast into inferior vena cava

   d. Right-sided segmental pulmonary embolism, dilated right ventricle and flattening of intraventricular septum, bilateral pleural effusions

   e. Right-sided segmental pulmonary embolism, infarction of the lung, dilated right ventricle, bilateral pleural effusions, hepatic congestion

The patient is referred to the acute internal medicine team and a bedside transthoracic echocardiogram is performed.

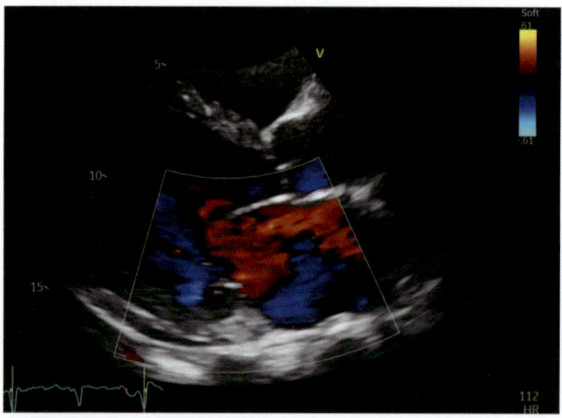

2. What is the main finding on the parasternal long axis view (PLAX) with colour flow Doppler?

   a. Tricuspid regurgitation

   b. Aortic regurgitation

   c. Aortic stenosis

   d. Mitral regurgitation

   e. Left atrial dilatation

The formal report of the transthoracic echo suggests an ejection fraction of 25% with severe RV, LV and biatrial dilatation. There is also evidence of pulmonary hypertension.

3.   What is the expectant median life expectancy of someone with these findings?

   a.   2 years

   b.   5 years

   c.   8 years

   d.   10 years

   e.   12 years

☑ 1c No large pulmonary embolism, dilated left ventricle, small pericardial effusion, bilateral pleural effusions, reflux of contrast into inferior vena cava

This CTPA shows a number of abnormalities. However, firstly we should assess for the primary indication, namely that of a pulmonary embolism. There is good opacification of the pulmonary vasculature as visualised by the bright white appearance of the contrast and there are no grey or black filling defects that would suggest a pulmonary embolism. Ensure to following the vasculature from the pulmonary trunk down to the subsegmental arteries. Then move on to assess the remainder of the scan for any other abnormalities. There is massive cardiomegaly with a significantly dilated left ventricle with a rim of pericardial fluid seen as a halo around the heart. There are bilateral pleural effusions, worse on the right. Lastly, looking closely, you may notice opacification of the inferior vena cava and hepatic veins; this is reflux of contrast media, which is suggestive of tricuspid regurgitation. In summary: no pulmonary embolism, large dilated heart with bilateral moderate pleural effusions with reflux of contrast into the inferior vena cava suggesting TR.

☑ 2d Mitral regurgitation

The left parasternal long axis view (PLAX) is achieved by placing the phased array transducer in the 3rd or 4th intercostal space on left sternal edge with patient lying on their left side with the transducer marker pointing towards patient's right shoulder. This view provides a good overview of left cardiac function and should give good visualisation of the left ventricle (LV) and left ventricular outflow tract (LVOT) along with a view of the aortic valve, left atrium, mitral valve, as well as the pericardium and descending thoracic aorta. You will get a glimpse of the right ventricle (RV), although it's generally a partial view. Colour flow Doppler allows visualisation of flow and velocity in a selected area – here over the mitral valve; flow away from the probe, negative Doppler shift, is visualised as blue; flow towards the probe, positive Doppler shift, is visualised as red (remember the mnemonic 'BART': **B**lue **A**way, **R**ed **T**owards). Flow can be seen backwards across the mitral valve during systole, suggesting mitral regurgitation.

☑ 3b 5 years

This gentleman has features suggestive of dilated cardiomyopathy (DCM) with evidence of decompensated heart failure. DCM is the most frequent form of primary myocardial disease and third most common cause of heart failure. Clinically, DCM is characterised by progressive course of ventricular dilatation and systolic dysfunction. The median survival time at point of diagnosis is approximately 5 years. Causes of DCM include ischaemic heart disease, hypertension, diabetes mellitus, HIV, viral hepatitis, myocarditis, alcohol, cocaine/amphetamine and anthracycline cytotoxics. Familial occurrence of DCM is believed to be responsible for 20–30% of cases and is mostly as an autosomal dominant trait with 24 genes identified. However, there is wide variability in onset, course and severity of the disease even within the same family.

KEY LEARNING POINTS

- When interpreting a CTPA for pulmonary emboli, look carefully through the arterial contrast phase for filling defects that will appear as hypoattenuating (black) areas.
- When using echocardiography to look at valvular function, colour Doppler provides a quick and easy way to look for relative velocity and flow patterns.
- Patients with dilated cardiomyopathy, in general, have a median survival rate of 5 years from diagnosis.

CASE 25

Epigastric pain

An 80-year-old woman presents to the emergency department with a 1-day history of generalised abdominal pain and reduced urine output. She has a history of hypertension, for which she takes atenolol and doxazosin. She lives alone and is fully independent of activities of daily living with an excellent quality of life.

Initial observations are recorded as HR 65, BP 68/50, SpO$_2$ 91% on room air, RR 20, temperature 36.7°C (98.1°F). On examination, she looks unwell, there is reduced air entry bibasally with no added sounds, the abdomen is soft with generalised tenderness on deep palpation, most marked in the epigastric region.

An ABG is performed, which reveals pH 7.23, pO$_2$ 7.7, pCO$_2$ 4.4, HCO$_3^-$ 18.2, BE –4.6, Lactate 3.9.

An erect chest radiograph is performed.

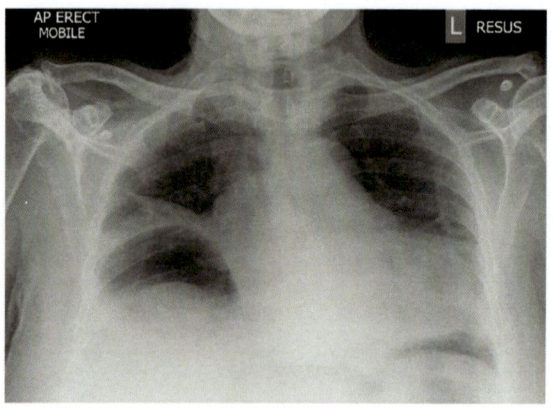

1. What is the most significant pathology visualised on the chest radiograph?

    a. Pneumoperitoneum

    b. Atelectasis

    c. Bilateral pleural effusions

    d. Distended bowel loops

    e. Bilateral lower lobe pneumonia

DOI: 10.1201/9781003461456-25

2. Based on your diagnosis, if the patient was haemodynamically stable, which imaging modality would you proceed to next?

    a. CT chest with oral and IV contrast

    b. Point-of-care eFAST ultrasound scan

    c. CT abdomen & pelvis with contrast

    d. Transthoracic echo

    e. Point-of-care thoracic ultrasound of the aorta

You review the laboratory bloods and note raised inflammatory markers with CRP 350 and WCC >20, and a stage 2 AKI with creatinine 128 and eGFR 22.

She has received 3 L IV balanced crystalloid solution in intermittent fluid boluses and remains hypotensive with a mean arterial pressure (MAP) of 50 mmHg.

3. Which of the following is the next best management plan?

    a. Broad-spectrum IV antibiotics to cover chest source and pleural aspiration

    b. Broad-spectrum IV antibiotics to cover abdominal source and refer for emergency surgical intervention

    c. High-flow nasal oxygen, IV furosemide for diuresis and referral to acute internal medicine team for consideration of CPAP

    d. Broad-spectrum antibiotics to cover abdominal source and referral to intensive care unit (ICU) for vasopressors

    e. Broad-spectrum antibiotics to cover abdominal source and further fluid resuscitation with colloid solution

☑ 1a Pneumoperitoneum

The most significant abnormality on this chest radiograph is gross pneumoperitoneum (gas within the peritoneal cavity) with raised hemidiaphragms bilaterally. If part of the clinical question for performing the chest radiograph is to exclude pneumoperitoneum, you must ensure the patient has been sitting up for around 10–15 minutes beforehand as air 'rises'. When assessing a chest radiograph, even if the abnormality is obvious, it is still important to review the rest of the radiograph in a systematic way to identify any other pathology. One such method is as follows: always start with patient identification and date of examination (removed in this image) and image quality (projection, rotation, inspiration and exposure), before a systematic check of anatomy. Anatomical structures to assess are trachea and bronchi, hilar structures, lung zones, pleura, lung lobes and fissures, costophrenic angles, diaphragm, heart, mediastinum, soft tissues and bones. We can see here that the gross pneumoperitoneum has led to bilateral lower lobe collapse, particularly prominent on the right side as the left is obscured by the cardiac shadow.

☑ 2c CT abdomen & pelvis with contrast

Alongside urgent referral to the general surgeons, if the patient is stable the best next step is to perform a CT abdomen & pelvis with contrast. This is because the most common cause of pneumoperitoneum is disruption of a hollow viscous, for example, peptic ulcer disease, bowel obstruction with perforation, perforated appendicitis, ischaemic bowel, traumatic perforation or iatrogenic perforation such as during colonoscopy. The CT will confirm the diagnosis and try to identify the site of perforation. If patient is unstable, they may require immediate transfer to theatre for emergency laparotomy. One benefit of point-of-care ultrasound scanning is it can be performed rapidly even in an unstable patient. However, though abdominal ultrasound can identify specific features that indicate free abdominal air, it is less able to identify the site of perforation. With regard to hypoxia in this case, it is most likely due to diaphragmatic splinting due to the gas and fluid within the peritoneal cavity, and reduced depth of breathing with secondary atelectasis due to pain. Do also remember that poor perfusion (shock) may lead to a less reliable pulse oximetry trace too.

☑ 3b Broad-spectrum IV antibiotics to cover abdominal source and emergency surgical intervention

Despite adequate fluid resuscitation, this woman remains hypotensive and therefore needs urgent surgical intervention to identify and repair the location of perforation. Note the patient has not mounted a tachycardia despite hypotension, likely secondary to her beta-blocker treatment. Broad-spectrum antibiotics according to local microbiology guidelines should be administered given the high suspicion of peritoneal soiling. Given the ongoing haemodynamic instability, she is likely to require vasopressor support pre- and intraoperatively and will require post-operative ICU admission. However, surgery should not be delayed for ICU review as ultimately the best management is repair of the perforation. Additionally, the anaesthetic team can liaise with ICU once the patient is in theatre for appropriate post-operative destination. This patient was taken to theatre urgently and found to have perforated duodenal ulcer with a large volume of free fluid in her abdomen. The perforation was repaired with an omental patch and she was transferred to ICU. Perforation affects up to 6% of patients who have peptic ulcer disease (PUD) and commonly presents in a similar fashion to this case with generalised acute abdominal pain, peritonism and shock. It is a surgical emergency and the majority of patients will undergo laparotomy and repair of the perforation. Risk factors for PUD include infection with *Helicobacter pylori*, non-steroidal anti-inflammatory drugs, corticosteroids, severe physiological stress and Zollinger–Ellison syndrome.

KEY LEARNING POINTS

- A systematic approach to chest radiograph interpretation will help identify all abnormalities and a simple approach is to assess the 'ABC' structures followed by 'Diagnostics' and 'Everything' else.
- CT abdomen & pelvis with contrast remains the gold standard for identifying sites of bowel perforation if the patient is physiologically stable.
- Early surgical and anaesthetic consultations are vital in tandem with broad-spectrum antibiotics and fluid resuscitation as patients may achieve excellent outcomes if co-morbidities are low.

CASE 26

Facial trauma

A 41-year-old man who is an ophthalmic surgeon is brought in by ambulance after a bicycle accident. He was cycling at 10 mph wearing a helmet, but lost balance on a bend and fell over the handlebars, landing on his face and outstretched hands.

Primary survey reveals no other significant injuries.

Facial views are requested.

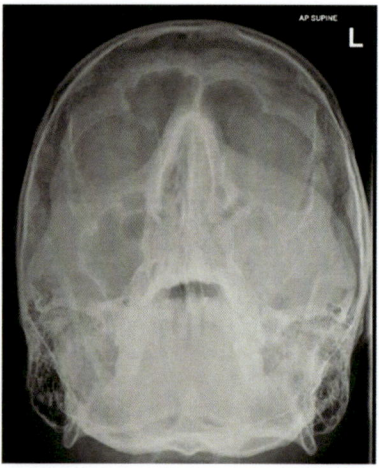

1. What are the major attachment points of the zygomatic complex to the facial skeleton?
   a. Frontozygomatic (F-Z) suture, orbital floor, maxillary sinus, zygomatic arch
   b. F-Z suture, zygomatic arch, zygomatic buttress, infraorbital rim
   c. Pterion, orbital floor, zygomatic arch, zygomatic buttress
   d. Pterion, greater wing of sphenoid, infraorbital rim, F-Z suture
   e. Zygomatic arch, greater wing of sphenoid, lacrimal bone, orbital floor

During assessment he complains of numbness in the left side of his upper lip and feels as if his upper incisors have been anaesthetised like he 'has been to the dentist'.

DOI: 10.1201/9781003461456-26

2. Which of the following best explains this phenomenon?

   a. Traumatic occlusion of the superior labial artery

   b. Maxillary sinus haematoma causing dental nerve root anaesthesia

   c. Zygomatic nerve injury

   d. Soft tissue oedema causing compression of neurovascular structures

   e. Infraorbital nerve injury

A CT of the facial bones is performed to assess the injury further.

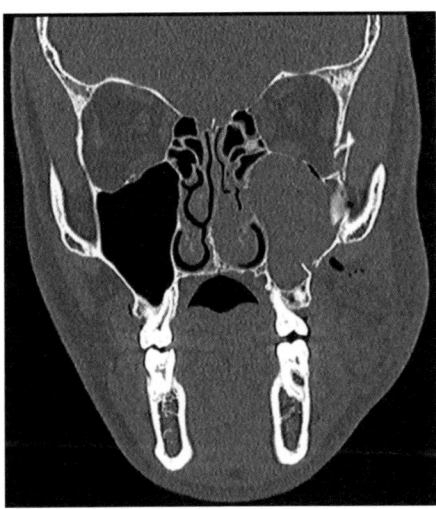

3. Which one of the following findings strongly suggests an orbital fracture?

   a. Diplopia on upward gaze

   b. Subconjunctival haemorrhage

   c. Eyelid laceration

   d. Traumatic mydriasis

   e. Hyphaema

☑ 1b Frontozygomatic suture, zygomatic arch, zygomatic buttress, infraorbital rim

A 'tripod fracture' (i.e. zygomaticomaxillary complex fracture) is one of the most common facial bone injuries seen after trauma. Appreciating the gross anatomy of the zygomatic complex helps identify the areas that are most at risk of injury. The term 'tripod' is somewhat of a misnomer; we can think of the zygomatic complex as having four legs that articulate with the frontal bone: the F-Z suture, the arch (with the temporal bone posterolaterally), the infraorbital rim medially and the buttress inferiorly. This plain film radiograph demonstrates fractures at all these sites in a classical pattern. The zygomatic complex carries important functions in the facial skeleton. Aside from acting as a site for muscle attachments and contributing to facial aesthetics, it provides protection of critical underlying structures such as the eye and the deep facial neurovasculature.

☑ 2e Infraorbital nerve injury

The most likely explanation for this pattern of altered sensation is a neuropraxic injury of the infraorbital nerve, a purely sensory nerve. The infraorbital nerve arises from the maxillary nerve (V2, second division of the trigeminal nerve) in the pterygopalatine fossa. It travels along the infraorbital groove of the orbital floor, where it is partially exposed. It gives off two to three dentoalveolar branches and, at its terminus, innervates the skin of the upper lip and paranasal skin. Orbital floor fractures frequently give rise to neuropraxic injury of this nerve. This can also happen with direct trauma to the tissue overlying the infraorbital foramen (from a front-facing blow, for example). A useful way to gauge the level of nerve injury is the presence of altered sensation to the upper incisors and gingivae. If present, this suggests injury within the orbit, as this is where the anterior superior alveolar branch is given off. The infraorbital nerve can be blocked by injection of local anaesthetic using an extraoral or intraoral approach with indications including anaesthesia for upper lip laceration repair, as well as analgesia for cleft lip surgical repair and surgery of the lower eyelid, median cheek and (septo)rhinoplasty. The most important technical aspect with either approach is to prevent penetration of the foramen to ensure the nerve is not damaged; this is achieved by keeping a finger on the foramen at all times throughout the procedure.

☑ 3a Diplopia on upward gaze

This CT shows a complex left sided facial bone complex injury – with the floor of the orbit, anterior and lateral walls of the maxillary sinus and zygoma fractured too. All of the listed options (diplopia, subconjunctival haemorrhage, eyelid laceration, hyphema, traumatic mydriasis) could suggest an orbital fracture but the most specific feature is diplopia on upward gaze. This would suggest entrapment of the inferior oblique muscle on the orbital floor with or without downward herniation of fat contents (classically seen as a teardrop on plain radiograph). Look carefully for subconjuctival haemorrhage which suggests either an orbital roof fracture or more commonly a base of skull fracture. Patients with these features should have CT scans of their head as well as their facial bones in this case to rule out intracranial bleeding. Most zygomaticomaxillary complex fractures can be managed expectantly with follow-up by maxillofacial surgeons in trauma clinics. However, in the presence of eye involvement (reduced visual acuity or diplopia), immediate referral to maxillofacial surgery and/or ophthalmology is required for urgent surgical intervention.

KEY LEARNING POINTS

- Plain facial bone radiographs are useful for screening for facial fractures. A good working knowledge of anatomy will help differentiate a fracture from suture lines.
- Clinical examination of mid-face fractures or injury should always include assessment of the infraorbital nerve, which is often injured.
- There are several signs that suggest an orbital fracture but diplopia on upward gaze is the most sensitive and specific for an orbital floor fracture with inferior oblique muscle entrapment.

Fall from a wheelchair

A 56-year-old woman, who is wheelchair bound, presents with shoulder pain after reporting that she was assaulted and pushed from her wheelchair. She is slightly challenging and does want you to examine her due to significant pain in her shoulder. She is known to have a history of illicit drug use but is limited in the further information she discloses.

You manage to convince her to have an radiograph following analgesia.

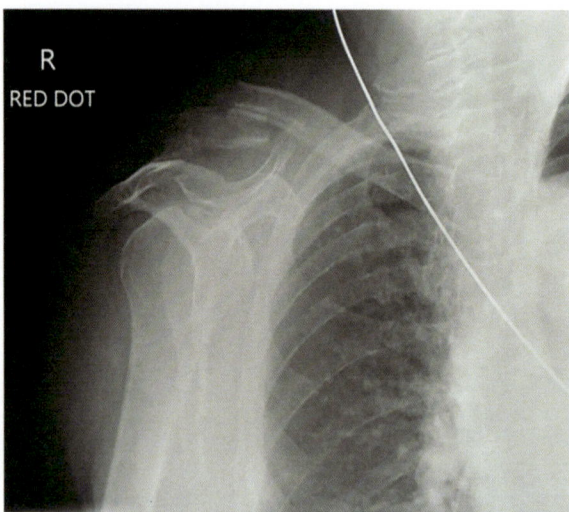

1. Based on the findings in the radiograph, which of the following is the best next step?

   a. Examine overlying skin, perform a sensorimotor examination and assess distal pulses

   b. Examine overlying skin, assess sensation in the hand and distal pulses and perform a 'cross-body test'

   c. Examine overlying skin, test capillary refill time and gross hand function

   d. Examine overlying skin, assess distal pulses, perform a sensorimotor examination and chest examination

   e. Examine overlying skin, test capillary refill time and perform a full elbow examination

DOI: 10.1201/9781003461456-27

2. Which structure(s) are most at risk with this pattern of injury?

   a. Brachial plexus and subclavian vessels

   b. Axillary artery and axillary nerve

   c. Scapular body and lung apex

   d. Brachial plexus and lung apex

   e. Proximal humerus

On examination there is no skin tenting or neurovascular compromise. You review an additional radiograph view.

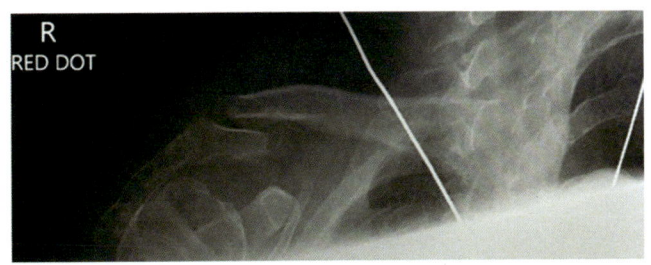

3. How are you going to proceed with the management of the injury in this patient?

   a. Apply a polysling, refer for physiotherapy assessment, follow-up in fracture clinic

   b. Apply a collar and cuff sling, discharge, follow-up in fracture clinic

   c. Refer to the orthopaedic team for consideration of surgical management

   d. Apply a high arm sling, discharge with no follow-up as she is unlikely to attend

   e. Refer to the orthopaedic team for admission due to mobility issues

☑ 1d Examine overlying skin, assess distal pulses, perform a sensorimotor examination and chest examination

Examination of the skin in patients with clavicular fractures often shows a slight visible bulge due to haematoma, but it is important to look carefully for tenting of the skin which suggests significant angulation and displacement. Tenting if left without intervention will lead to skin necrosis. Other potential complications associated with this injury pattern include compression of the subclavian vessels and brachial plexus injury. A thorough neurovascular examination should be undertaken including skin colour, distal pulses and a detailed sensorimotor examination of the upper limb to exclude these. Remember that assessing capillary refill time alone may miss a vascular injury. The 'cross-body test' involves adduction of the arm horizontally across the chest bringing the elbow towards the opposite shoulder; a positive test reproduces pain localised over the acromioclavicular joint. However, it is positive for both acromioclavicular joint separations and fractures of the lateral third of the clavicle and therefore is not a discriminator. One should also examine the chest, particularly if the injury is of high velocity or, as in this case, bone quality is poor, to exclude additional injuries such as rib fractures, scapula fractures and haemothorax and/or pneumothorax. There are old, healed rib fractures on this radiograph.

☑ 2a Brachial plexus and subclavian vessels

Due to their close relation, as mentioned above, lateral third clavicular fractures are associated with a small risk of acute injury to underlying subclavian vessels and the brachial plexus. Subclavian vessel injury is a rare consequence and most often is due to penetrating trauma. However, damage to the subclavian artery following clavicular fracture secondary to blunt trauma is possible with bone fragments leading to stretching, transection or compression of the vessel. Although the brachial plexus is also at risk in lateral third clavicular fractures, this would commonly present with a nerve trunk palsy, rather than injury of a specific branch and so this excludes axillary artery and nerve. Pneumothorax can occur due to injury at the lung apex but this and haemothorax are more commonly associated with fractures of the medial third of the clavicle. Scapular fractures are rare, with the majority caused by high energy trauma such as road traffic collisions; they are commonly associated with other traumatic injuries including thoracic injury, fractures of ribs/clavicle/spine, pelvic and other extremity injury.

☑ 3c Refer to the orthopaedic team for consideration of surgical management

Indications for orthopaedic referral for patients with clavicular fracture include: open fractures, evidence of skin tenting, neurovascular compromise, comminuted fractures and significant medialisation (>2 cm if aged 12 years or over). This second radiograph view highlights the significant medialisation of the lateral fragment that warrants orthopaedic assessment within the emergency department due to high risk of malunion or non-union; with conservative management this can be as high as 30–40%. The argument for urgent surgical fixation is even more compelling as this patient relies on the use of both arms for her wheelchair. Lateral third clavicle fractures are often fixed with a plate and screws. Other advantages of surgical management alongside higher union rates and faster time to union include improved functional outcomes and cosmetic satisfaction. Disadvantages of surgical management include risk of symptomatic hardware, loss of fixation and/or migration of metalwork, risk of need for future procedures, paraesthesia and dysmorphic scar.

KEY LEARNING POINTS

- Plain radiographs are often sufficient to diagnose a clavicle fracture; however, remember to look for associated injuries such as rib fractures, pneumothoraces or scapula fractures.
- Remember to perform a screening neurovascular examination in all patients pre-senting with an upper limb or clavicle injury to look for possible brachial plexus injury.
- Patient handedness, occupation and special needs such as wheelchair use may influence treatment choice when deciding between non-operative and operative management.

Fall in the playground

A 4-year-old girl presents to the emergency department with her parents, complaining of left arm pain. She was playing in a playground 1 hour ago and was witnessed to trip whilst running, falling onto her outstretched hand. There was no head injury and she cried straight away. Her mother and father took her home first but noted she was reluctant to move the arm despite giving a dose of ibuprofen. There is no other medical history of note, and she is fully immunised. The mother tells you that she is mostly right-handed.

On examination, she is reluctant to move the left arm at all and you note a tender swollen elbow. Screening examination of the hand, wrist, forearm and shoulder is normal. This appears to be a closed injury and the hand is warm and well perfused.

You are about to perform a neurovascular exam and remember an easy way to test motor function with the game 'rock, paper, scissors, OK'.

1. Which of the following are the correct action and nerve pairings?
    a. Rock – median nerve, paper – radial nerve, scissors – ulnar nerve
    b. Rock – radial nerve, paper – ulnar nerve, scissors – median nerve
    c. Rock – ulnar nerve, paper – median nerve, scissors – radial nerve
    d. Rock – median nerve, paper – radial nerve, scissors – anterior interosseous nerve
    e. Rock – median nerve, paper – anterior interosseous nerve, scissors – ulnar nerve

You document a pain score of 6/10, prescribe the appropriate dose of paracetamol according to patient age, and order radiographs of the left elbow.

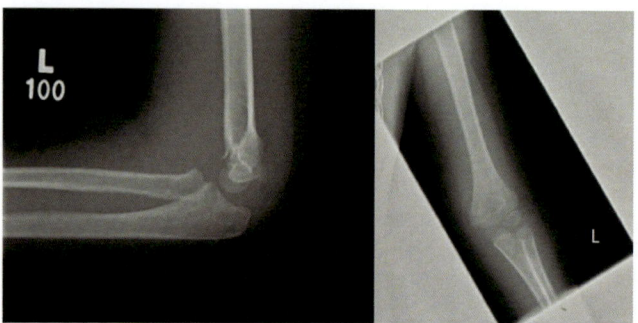

DOI: 10.1201/9781003461456-28

2. Which of the following ossification centres would you expect to see in a child of this age from this list?

    a. Internal epicondyle

    b. Trochlear

    c. Olecranon

    d. Capitellum

    e. External epicondyle

You compare the radiographs to a commonly used classification system for paediatric elbow fractures; it appears to correspond to a Gartland Grade II injury.

3. Which of the following best describes how would you treat this injury?

    a. Place in a broad arm sling, advise it can be removed at night and discharge with advice to return if it does not settle in a week

    b. Place in a removable wrist brace with thumb extension and refer to hand fracture clinic

    c. Apply an above elbow backslab and refer to orthopaedics for consideration of manipulation under anaesthesia

    d. Apply a U-slab and refer for follow-up in fracture clinic

    e. Apply a collar and cuff sling and refer for follow-up in fracture clinic

☑ 1a Rock – median nerve, paper – radial nerve, scissors – ulnar nerve

In addition, 'OK' = anterior interosseous nerve (AIN), which is a branch of the median nerve that may be injured in forearm fractures. A thorough neurovascular assessment is essential as part of any musculoskeletal injury assessment, and it is frequently documented inadequately. It is key to assess both the motor and sensory function of each nerve that may pass through the region of injury and provide clear documentation of such assessment. When assessing the hand, a rapid way of testing sensation is to assess the 'principal' area. There can be variation in the sensory supply to the hand, but the principal areas are always supplied as follows: median nerve – palmar surface of the index finger; ulnar nerve – palmar surface of the little finger; and radial nerve – first dorsal web space. The same should be done with the incoming vascular supply in the form of pulses and tissue perfusion (capillary refill time). In both children and adults, 'rock, paper, scissors, OK', represents a fun and simple way of assessing the motor function to the hand as it is familiar to both patient and clinician and relies on simple language.

☑ 2d Capitellum

The elbow radiograph in a child can be challenging to interpret due to the presence of ossification centres which fuse at various ages. The order of these can be remembered by a simple mnemonic of CRITOE (1, 3, 5, 7, 9, 11 years): **C**apitellum (1), **R**adial head (3), **I**nternal epicondyle (5), **T**rochlear (7), **O**lecranon (9), **E**xternal epicondyle (11). In a child of 4 years, you would expect to see the capitellum *and* radial head centres. There are a number of other aspects to look through in a systemic manner before the ossification centres. Firstly, look at the lateral view for the presence of a 'fat pad'. This represents a joint effusion, and the presence of a posterior fat pad is always abnormal. A small anterior one can be normal, but if large, this suggests an intra-articular injury. Next consider the 'anterior humeral line', which is a line drawn down the anterior cortex of the humerus. This should pass through the middle third of the capitellum and is disrupted in a supracondylar fracture. Next, look at the 'radio-capitellar' line, which should pass through the middle of the proximal end of the radius and bisect the capitellum in both lateral and anterior-posterior (AP) views. Disruption suggests a dislocation of the radial head. Then, look at the angle of the radial head for subtle angulation that may indicate a fracture and the cortex lines of the distal humerus on anterior and posterior borders. You should be able to identify a posterior fat pad, disruption of the anterior humeral line and supracondylar fracture in the lateral view. The AP view is less helpful, but here you can see a subtle supracondylar fracture.

☑ 3c Apply an above elbow backslab and refer to orthopaedics for consideration of manipulation under anaesthesia

Supracondylar fractures are graded by the Gartland system, which classifies them into three grades depending on degree of displacement on the lateral view: Grade I – both cortices of the distal humerus are breached but undisplaced; Grade II – both cortices breached, posterior tilt but intact posterior cortex; Grade III – both cortices breached and severe displacement. Grade I can be managed conservatively in an above elbow cast and fracture clinic, Grade II may need manipulation under anaesthesia and plaster of Paris, and Grade III needs operative intervention with manipulation under anaesthesia +/– insertion of K-wires before immobilisation in plaster of Paris. In this case with a Grade II injury, specialist input was sought from the orthopaedic team, and the fracture managed conservatively with an above elbow cast for 3 weeks, before removal and active mobilisation. If in doubt, get specialist or senior advice as correct healing is critical to onward function and the restoration of full extension in the child.

KEY LEARNING POINTS

- A complete neurovascular assessment should be clearly documented for musculoskeletal injuries; 'rock, paper, scissors, OK' is useful for children and adults.
- Ossification centres in the elbow develop according to age of the child and can make the radiographs confusing to interpret.
- Grade II and III supracondylar fractures should be referred for specialist review to ensure no functional impairment occurs due to incorrect healing.

Fever and back pain

A 64-year-old man presents to the emergency department with a history of lower back pain for the last week. He was seen in urgent treatment centre a few days earlier and discharged with a diagnosis of 'mechanical' pain. He now describes difficulty opening his bowels and urinary incontinence in the last 2 days, with a complete inability to mobilise due to bilateral leg pain which is slightly worse on the right. He has also been feeling hot and clammy intermittently. He has a past medical history of psoriasis. He works as a security officer, is 198 cm tall and weighs 180 kg.

Initial observations are recorded as HR 101, BP 168/72, SpO_2 97% on room air, RR 20, temperature 37.8°C (100.0°F). On focused neurological examination of the lower limbs, he is lying on a trolley and unable to mobilise due to pain, tone is normal bilaterally, power MRC 3+/5 hip flexion, 4/5 hip extension, 4/5 knee flexion and extension, 4/5 ankle dorsiflexion and plantarflexion, 5/5 great toe dorsiflexion.

1. Which of the following is the best imaging modality to confirm or exclude the top differential diagnoses?
   a. CT lumbosacral spine
   b. MRI lumbosacral spine
   c. No imaging indicated at this stage
   d. Radiograph lumbosacral spine
   e. Ultrasound abdomen

A digital rectal examination is performed with normal anal tone and perianal sensation. A post-void bladder scan shows 50 mL residual.

You review the blood results and note WCC 14.06, CRP 376, normal renal and liver function.

Despite assistance from the radiographers, the patient is too large for the primary imaging modality.

DOI: 10.1201/9781003461456-29

An alternative is performed.

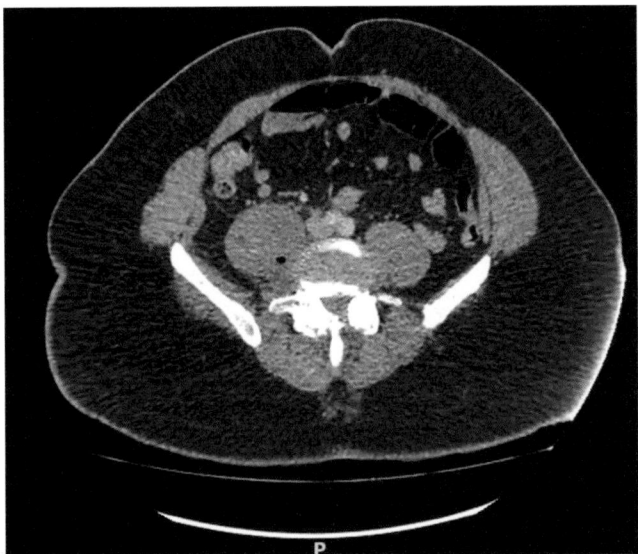

2. Which of the following is the best description of the displayed scan?

    a. Psoas abscess

    b. Acute cholecystitis with pericolic abscess

    c. Lumbar spondylodiscitis

    d. Acute appendicitis with abscess

    e. Acute pyelonephritis

3. What is the most common organism implicated with this condition?

    a. *Streptococcus pyogenes*

    b. *Bacteroides fragilis*

    c. *Mycobacterium tuberculosis*

    d. *Staphylococcus aureus*

    e. *Escherichia coli*

☑ 1b MRI lumbosacral spine

The main differential diagnosis in this case is cauda equina syndrome (suggested by lower back pain, bilateral leg pain and difficulty in voiding). However, the added complication in this case is the fever which hints at infection complicating the matter. When assessing a patient with back pain, remember the red flag symptoms that warrant investigation include bowel/bladder dysfunction, progressive motor weakness, saddle anaesthesia, bilateral radiculopathy/sciatica, laxity of the anal sphincter, erectile dysfunction, severe night pain, unexplained weight loss, fever, history of tuberculosis or HIV or an individual who is immunocompromised. MRI is the imaging modality of choice for patients with lower back pain and red flags suggestive of cauda equina syndrome, but CT with contrast can be used in patients when MRI is contraindicated or unavailable. Plain radiographs have limited value in assessing suspected cauda equina syndrome. Ultrasound abdomen would be indicated if acute cholecystitis were suspected but may be technically challenging in this patient due to the patient's body habitus. Prior to imaging, an initial assessment of the patient should follow the standard ABCDE method as this provides a rapid screen through the main body systems to identify any abnormalities including potential sites of infection. Bloods should be drawn including FBC, U&Es, CRP, coagulation screen, blood cultures and urine sample taken for dipstick testing and microscopy & culture. It would be prudent to cover the patient with broad-spectrum antibiotics according to local microbiology guidelines once cultures have been taken. Have a low threshold to catheterise the patient as this will provide a measure of renal function and decompress and protect the bladder if cauda equina syndrome is proven.

☑ 2a Psoas abscess

The striking abnormality is the enlarged psoas muscle on the right with the presence of gas locules. Review the cine loop again at around 01m03s. This is characteristic of a psoas abscess and would explain the patient's symptoms of worsening back pain and fever. Note the size of the patient's forearms on the CT! Considering the other diagnoses, the gallbladder here appears to be normal and devoid of stones. Remember that not all gallstones are CT opaque and hence ultrasound scan is recommended if the CT is normal. Features of spondylodiscitis include disc space narrowing with irregularity of the vertebral endplates as well as surrounding soft tissue swelling and intervertebral disc enhancement. There is no perinephric fat stranding to suggest acute pyelonephritis. This appears as 'streaking' in the fat surrounding the kidney and again compare one side to the other if looking for this sign specifically. Although the pelvis is crowded, the appendix is visualised and not inflamed and there is no fat stranding in the surrounding mesentery making acute appendicitis unlikely.

☑ 3d *Staphylococcus aureus*

A psoas abscess can be primary or secondary in origin: primary being haematogenous or lymphatic seeding from a distant infection and secondary being as a result of direct spread of infection to the psoas muscle from an adjacent structure. Risk factors for primary abscess include diabetes mellitus, intravenous drug use, HIV, renal failure and other forms of immunosuppression; trauma leading to psoas haematoma formation can also be a risk factor. Adjacent structures involved in secondary abscesses may include the vertebral bodies and discs, the hip joint, the gastrointestinal tract (appendix), the genitourinary tract, vascular structures and other sites. The most common organism isolated is *Staphylococcus aureus* (90% of cases) and the history of psoriasis is relevant here as it may provide a portal of entry for bacteria. Don't forget to test for HIV should local availability allow. Psoas abscesses are commonly missed or diagnosed late due to the non-specific initial symptoms. Management includes administration of antibiotics and consideration of drainage of the abscess (image-guided or surgically), particularly if the abscess is large and/or multiloculated.

KEY LEARNING POINTS

- Think of infections such as discitis or psoas abscess in cases of true back pain in the presence of fever.
- MRI gives best visualisation of soft tissues including discs but CT with contrast can be considered if technical factors preclude MRI.
- *Staphylococcus aureus* is the most common causative agent for a psoas abscess and the mainstay of treatment is high dose flucloxacillin antibiotics and CT-guided drainage if the abscess collection is large.

CASE 30

Fever in a returning traveller

A 44-year-old man presents to the emergency department (ED) complaining of 2 days of intermittent fever, associated with abdominal pain and headaches not improving with paracetamol. He has recently moved to London after 15 years living in Lagos, Nigeria. He does not have any other medical conditions and does not take any regular medications.

Initial observations are recorded as HR 110, BP 148/83, SpO_2 98% on room air, RR 22, temperature 38.8°C (101.8°F). On examination, he is alert and orientated. He is sweating profusely. Respiratory and cardiovascular examinations are normal, but he complains of tenderness in the right upper quadrant on palpation of the abdomen.

The laboratory phones to inform you that his platelet count is 70 and a blood film is being performed.

The initial film is shown.

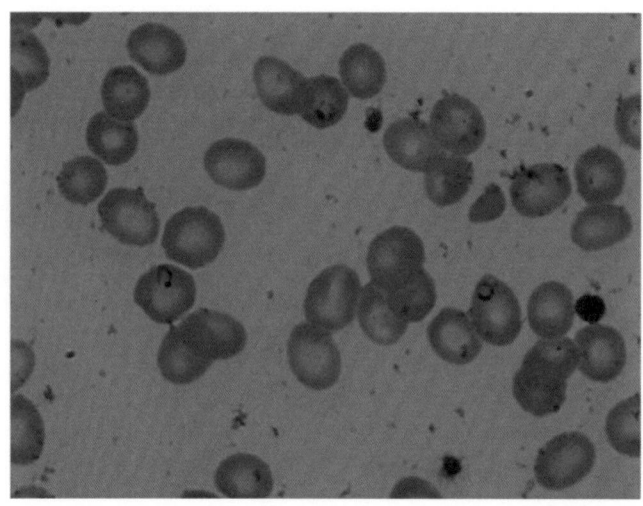

DOI: 10.1201/9781003461456-30

1. What is the likely diagnosis and associated blood film finding?

    a. Sleeping sickness – African *Trypanosoma mastigotes*

    b. Vivax malaria – *Plasmodium vivax* ring stage

    c. Babesiosis – *Babesia microti* ring form

    d. Knowlesi malaria – *Plasmodium knowlesi* hypnozoites

    e. Falciparum malaria – *Plasmodium falciparum* ring stage

The parasitology laboratory calls and confirms your diagnosis. The parasite count is 1.2% with early schizonts visible on the blood film.

On review, the patient's repeat observations are HR 94, BP 143/79, SpO$_2$ 98% on room air, RR 20, temperature 39°C (102.2°F). The chest is clear to auscultation but there is persistent pain in the right upper quadrant of the abdomen. He remains alert with GCS 15/15. Capillary blood glucose is 6.3 mmol/L.

The patient is referred to the infectious diseases team, which accepts him for admission.

2. Which one of the following features is most consistent with the risk of severe disease?

    a. Parasite count 1.2%

    b. Schizonts on blood film

    c. Fever 39°C

    d. Platelets 70

    e. Right upper quadrant pain

The infectious diseases registrar asks you to commence immediate treatment in the ED. You note liver function tests are mildly deranged (mild transaminitis). He weighs 90 kg.

Whilst checking the patient's drug allergies, he tells you that he is very allergic to a drug that he had in Nigeria for a similar presentation that made him 'itch' all over.

3. Which of the following is the best option to prescribe for this patient?

    a. Pentamidine: 360 mg IV or IM

    b. Azithromycin: 500 mg PO

    c. Quinine: 20 mg/kg (max 1.4 g) IV in 5% dextrose over 4 hours with cardiac and capillary blood glucose monitoring

    d. Artesunate: 220 mg IV (2.4 mg/kg)

    e. Quinine: 600 mg TDS PO for 5 days plus doxycycline 200 mg OD PO for 7 days

☑ 1e Falciparum malaria – *Plasmodium falciparum* ring stage

A suspected diagnosis of falciparum malaria can be made based on clinical features and recent travel from a high-risk area for exposure to *Plasmodium falciparum*. *P. falciparum* classically forms a fine ring with either a single or double chromatin dot in its ring stage and is responsible for >90% of malaria cases in Nigeria. In contrast, *P. vivax* forms an amoeboid shape and is conspicuously absent from Nigeria (<1% of cases). *P. knowlesi* is not found in Africa; it is endemic to South-East Asia and is thought to be zoonosis crossing from macaques. Sleeping sickness is a tropical disease caused by parasitic protozoans that are transmitted by the tsetse fly and presents with non-specific signs in early stages such as fever, headaches, lymphadenopathy and arthralgia. It later progresses to altered behaviour, confusion, sensory disturbance and sleep-wake disturbance, which gives it its name. Characteristic large worm-like flagellate organisms outside the red blood cells may be seen on blood smear. Babesia, a tick-borne parasite in the USA, may mimic malaria ring forms. The presence of tetrad merozoites (Maltese crosses) on the blood film is pathognomic.

☑ 2b Schizonts on blood film

Malaria is the most commonly imported tropical disease to the UK with approximately three-quarters of cases caused by *P. falciparum*. The feature here suggestive in this case of severe or complicated falciparum malaria is schizonts on the blood film as this is associated with a poorer prognosis. Other indications of severe malaria that are not present here are: parasitaemia >10%, severe anaemia (Hb <80), acidosis (pH <7.3), impaired consciousness or seizures, hypoglycaemia (<2.2 mmol/L), pulmonary oedema, renal impairment, haemoglobinuria, spontaneous bleeding or DIC and haemodynamic shock. The UK malaria treatment guidelines indicate all patients with falciparum malaria should be admitted initially regardless of clinical state due to the risk of deterioration. However, some specialist units that see a large volume of patients may ambulate those with uncomplicated falciparum malaria and low parasite loads. Patients who are clinically well with non-falciparum malaria are usually treated on an outpatient basis.

☑ 3d Artesunate: 220 mg IV (2.4 mg/kg)

Treatment of severe or complicated falciparum malaria requires urgent parenteral anti-malarials to have the biggest impact on prognosis. Evidence shows that intravenous artesunate is more efficacious that intravenous quinine, and therefore this is the treatment of choice in severe disease. Note that artesunate is not licensed in the European Union, but it is stocked by many specialist infectious diseases units in the UK. The suggested dosing schedule is 2.4 mg/kg IV bolus at 0, 12, 24 hours and then once-daily dosing. If artesunate is not immediately available or if working in other centres, treatment should not be delayed until it can be obtained. Intravenous quinine dihydrochloride is an alternative with the initial loading dose being 20 mg/kg (maximum 1.4 g) infused over 4 hours followed by 10 mg/kg (maximum 700 mg) every 8 hours. Note that the loading dose should not be given if the patient has received quinine or mefloquine in the previous 12 hours. The major side effects are hypoglycaemia, prolonged QTc (caution in cardiac disease) and itching in some patients of African descent. The pruritis can often be managed symptomatically but for a small minority of patients, it can be very severe. Also remember to reduce the dose of quinine by 30% in hepatic impairment. Oral quinine plus doxycycline is one option for the treatment of uncomplicated falciparum malaria. Pentamidine is the treatment of choice for African trypanosomiasis (sleeping sickness), while azithromycin is an option in babesiosis.

KEY LEARNING POINTS

- Malaria remains one of the most frequent treatable imported illnesses in the UK.
- Screening should be routinely performed in patients returning from endemic areas with a history of episodic fever, even if treatment was administered abroad.
- Remember to look for additional risk factors for severe malaria even if parasite loads appear to be low on peripheral blood films.
- Artesunate is rapidly replacing quinine as first-line treatment for falciparium malaria due to its effectiveness although resistance is emerging.

CASE 31

Haemoptysis and a swelling

A 41-year-old man presents to the emergency department with haemoptysis. He states he has had small amounts of blood-streaked sputum for the past couple of weeks, but today he had coughed up approximately 'a cup' of bright red blood. He has always lived in the UK and has no unwell contacts. He denies any weight loss. On systematic review, he tells you that he has been suffering from a painless scrotal swelling for which he is awaiting an outpatient urology appointment.

Initial observations are recorded as HR 86, BP 121/57, SpO$_2$ 99% on room air, RR 18, temperature 36.6°C (97.9°F). He looks comfortable at rest. Chest auscultation reveals good air entry bilaterally with scattered crackles bilaterally. The abdomen is soft and non-tender but genital examination reveals a large, grapefruit-sized, scrotal swelling on the right.

Bloods are drawn for venous blood gas (VBG), FBC, U&Es, CRP and coagulation profile.

1. Which of the following additional initial investigations should be ordered?

   a. Sputum MC&S, urine dipstick, chest radiograph

   b. D-dimer, sputum MC&S and AFB smear & culture, urine dipstick, chest radiograph

   c. Group & screen, urine dipstick, chest radiograph

   d. Group & screen, D-dimer, sputum MC&S and AFB smear & culture, chest radiograph

   e. Autoimmune screen, blood cultures, sputum MC&S, chest radiograph

Whilst waiting for the blood results, a chest radiograph is performed.

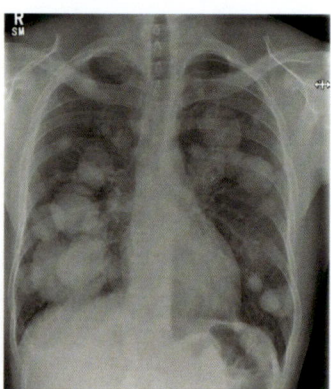

DOI: 10.1201/9781003461456-31

2. Given the above, which of the following blood tests would you add for this patient?

    a. PSA, LDH, AFP

    b. PSA, LDH, hCG

    c. LDH, hCG, AFP

    d. PSA, LDH, hCG, HE4

    e. PSA, LDH, hCG, AFP

The patient is referred to the acute internal medical team for further investigation and speciality team input.

As part of the work-up, the patient undergoes a CT abdomen & pelvis with contrast.

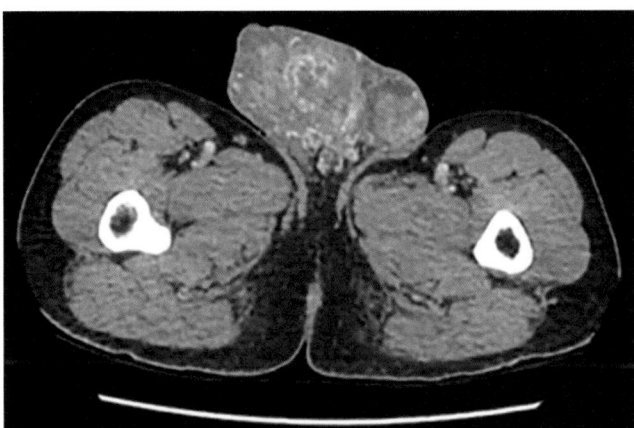

3. Which of the following is the best unifying diagnosis?

    a. Renal cell carcinoma (RCC) with lung metastases

    b. Prostate carcinoma with lung metastases

    c. Primary lung carcinoma with testicular metastases

    d. Testicular cancer with lung metastases

    e. Cancer of unknown primary (CUP)

☑ 1a Sputum MC&S, urine dipstick, chest radiograph

This patient presented to department with frank haemoptysis and the differential here is wide. Considering the causes of haemoptysis, the broad causes could be grouped as infection (for example, bacterial pneumonia especially cavitating types, tuberculosis, aspergilloma), pulmonary embolism, underlying lung disease (for example, bronchiecta-sis), autoimmune (for example, Churg–Strauss syndrome), cancer (primary lung malig-nancy or metastases), foreign bodies or trauma. It is tempting to send lots of additional blood tests including D-dimer and autoimmune screen at this stage to begin to investi-gate some of these potential differentials, but this may cloud the water and indeed the diagnosis. The best approach would be to take a detailed history, examine the patient thoroughly and alongside the basic blood set send a urine test due to the scrotal swelling and of course, a chest radiograph. As this is not massive haemoptysis, a group & screen test is not required as yet. Additionally, always consider that this could be pseudohae-moptysis (bleeding from a source other than the lower respiratory tract), which can be due to haematemesis aspirated into the lungs, bleeding from posterior nasal passage or nasopharynx or upper airway that can stimulate a cough reflex or material that is expectorated that looks like blood but is not, for example, *Serratia marcescens* infection.

☑ 2e PSA, LDH, hCG, AFP

The chest film shows multiple large, well-circumscribed, round shaped pulmonary masses. These are commonly called 'cannonball' metastases. When we see cannon-ball metastases, think of the mnemonic 'CRESP', which stands for: **C**: choriocarcinoma (a subtype of testicular or ovarian germ cell tumours (GCTs) or gestational trophoblastic disease), **R**: RCC, **E**: endometrial carcinoma, **S**: synovial sarcoma (soft tissue tumours affecting young patients and most commonly the tissue around the knees), **P**: pros-tate carcinoma. In the context of history of scrotal swelling and cannonball pulmonary metastases, the most likely diagnosis from the above would be a testicular GCT. When dealing with testicular GCTs, tumour markers can help to identify which subtype may be present and guide disease management. The three commonest tumour markers are alpha fetoprotein (AFP), human chorionic gonadotropin (hCG) and lactate dehydrogenase (LDH). In addition to the GCT tumour markers, ordering PSA would be reasonable, given the fact that prostate cancers might cause lymphoedema and swelling in the scrotum.

☑ 3d Testicular cancer with lung metastases

The striking abnormality captured on this CT is the scrotal swelling with solid intra-scro-tal masses. In this absence of bowel loops, this is not an inguinoscrotal hernia. The renal outlines are normal and so this is not an RCC and the liver appears to be free of masses too. The unifying diagnosis is therefore testicular cancer with pulmonary metastases. Testicular cancer tends to affect men between 15 and 49 years of age. Increased risk may be associated with undescended testes, a family history of cancer, Caucasians and smoking. The most common type of cancer is germ cell testicular cancer, which accounts for >95% of all cases. There are two main subtypes: seminomas (most common) and non-seminomas (teratoma, choriocarcinomas, yolk sac tumours). Management for all cases includes orchidectomy, followed by chemotherapy. A short course of radiotherapy may be recommended in some instances. The keys to early diagnosis in testicular cancer are self-examination and early referral for specialist assessment of scrotal masses.

KEY LEARNING POINTS

- Initial investigations should be chosen to be as high yield as possible to either rule in or rule out diagnoses and tailored by good history-taking and clinical examination.
- The most common causes of testicular cancer in young men are seminomas. The mainstay of treatment is orchidectomy and adjuvant chemotherapy.
- Only send tumour markers when you have a good working diagnosis. Urinary β-HCG levels can be tested for using a standard pregnancy dipstick. It is secreted by some germ cell and non-germ cell tumours and may help to confirm the diagnosis in the ED. A negative result does not exclude a testicular cancer.

Headache with lethargy

A 27-year-old woman attends the emergency department with intractable severe global headache that has come on gradually over the past 4 days with associated nausea and lethargy. She has no fever or cough, but a family member was unwell with coryzal symptoms a week ago. She has no past medical history and takes no regular medications. She is a non-smoker, lives with her husband and two children at home and works as a waitress. She occasionally suffers with headaches, but this is much worse than ever before.

Initial observations are all within normal limits. Focused neurological examination, including cranial nerve examination is normal.

1. Which of the following investigations would you request at this stage?
    a. Perform fundoscopy, draw blood for FBC/U&Es/CRP
    b. This is likely a tension-type headache and she doesn't need any investigations
    c. Draw blood for FBC/U&Es/CRP
    d. Perform fundoscopy, draw blood for FBC/U&Es/CRP/coagulation profile, urinary β-hCG, request non-contrast CT head
    e. Request contrast CT head

The investigations performed are reportedly 'normal' and do not seem to show any explanation for the cause of her symptoms. On further review she mentions that both her husband and children are also quite lethargic and have been complaining of abdominal pain. She has done very few shifts at work recently but no-one else has been unwell there.

2. Which test might hold the key in light of this further information?
    a. Venous blood gas (VBG)
    b. Repeat CT head with contrast in the venous phase
    c. Urine dipstick and pregnancy test
    d. Vitals signs: BP, RR, SpO_2, blood glucose
    e. Full blood count

DOI: 10.1201/9781003461456-32

3. Based on the suspected diagnosis, what treatment or investigation should be offered?

    a. Lumbar puncture for CSF sampling and examination

    b. High-flow oxygen therapy, screen family, call emergency gas services

    c. Coagulation and dilute Russell viper venom time

    d. Intravenous sodium thiosulphate

    e. High-flow oxygen therapy, intravenous hydroxocobalamin

☑ 1d Perform fundoscopy, draw blood for FBC/U&Es/CRP/ coagulation profile, urinary bHCG, request non-contrast CT head

The first step in all patients presenting with headache is to take a careful history of pain, for example by use of the mnemonic SOCRATES (**S**ite, **O**nset, **C**haracter, **R**adiation, **A**lleviation, **T**ime course, **E**xacerbation, **S**everity). Additionally, remember to ask questions that look at the relationship of the headache to other things such as reading, movement, exercise, vision, trauma and an environmental or occupational cause. Clinical examination should include vital signs, in particular BP, visual acuity, fundoscopy and capillary blood glucose in all cases. The key warning sign here is that the headaches are substantially different to normal. Other red flags include sudden-onset headache reaching maximum intensity in 5 minutes, presence of increasing headache with fever, new neurological deficit/cognitive dysfunction, headache triggered by cough/Valsalva/ exercise, headache that changes with posture and symptoms suggestive of giant cell arteritis or acute narrow angle glaucoma. In patients with headaches that are worse with position, consider a CT venogram to rule out central venous sinus thrombosis (CVST) particularly if the D-dimer is raised.

☑ 2a Venous blood gas (VBG)

A tricky case but the clues are there; primarily the fact that the family members are affected suggests an environmental cause at home. The unifying diagnosis here is carbon monoxide poisoning. Carboxyhaemoglobin (COHb) levels are displayed on the VBG results, though often this value is overlooked. Normal COHb levels are 1–3% for non-smokers, up to 5% in pregnancy or anaemia, up to 10–13% in smokers. With regard to the other options and what the abnormality might indicate: FBC – assessing for severe anaemia; urine dipstick and urinary β-hCG – to look for glycosuria, protein and pregnancy; CT head with contrast – acute bleed, space occupying lesion (sometimes missed on non-contrast scans) and hydrocephalus; vitals to look for hypertensive crisis and atypical hyperglycaemic crisis. Features of carbon monoxide poisoning depend on the level of exposure. Brief exposure to low levels can cause headache, dizziness, nausea and vomiting, flushing and muscle pains; exposure to higher levels can cause confusion, movement disorders, myocardial infarction, loss of consciousness and even death. Chronic exposure to low levels can cause headache, lethargy, nausea, visual disturbance, memory and neuropsychiatric problems. If symptoms are suggestive of carbon monoxide poisoning, also ask if anyone else at home is affected, if symptoms improve when out of the house, if fuel burning appliances and vents are maintained, and if they have a carbon monoxide alarm.

☑ 3b High-flow oxygen therapy, screen family, call emergency gas services

Based on the suspected diagnosis of carbon monoxide poisoning, the correct treatment is high-flow oxygen delivered by a tight-fitting mask. COHb levels rapidly decline and a repeat VBG in 30 minutes should show a considerable drop. In terms of key values, COHb 15–20% are clinically symptomatic and COHb 30% indicates severe poisoning. This patient had a COHb level of 26% on arrival. Do not forget to screen other family members and find the offending appliance. Most properties do have a carbon monoxide monitor installed now but they are only good if maintained appropriately. In terms of the alternative options, lumbar puncture would be indicated for suspected subarachnoid haemorrhage if CT is negative, sodium thiosulphate and hydroxocobalamin are treatments for cyanide poisoning in fire entrapment, dilute Russell viper venom time screens for lupus anticoagulant in systemic lupus erythematosus (SLE).

KEY LEARNING POINTS

- Careful and repeated history-taking can sometimes hold the key to complex cases. Ask about the health of dependents and partners as this might unveil a clue.
- Carbon monoxide poisoning is rapidly detected on venous blood gas samples and the level correlates to severity of exposure.
- Most countries will have dedicated safety reporting mechanisms (National Gas Emergency Service, UK), as well as governmental agencies (Health and Safety Executive Gas Safety Advice Line, UK). Ensure that patients and their families do not return until instructed to do so by the fire emergency services and gas safety team.

CASE 33

High fevers in a child

A 7-year-old boy presents to the emergency department with his mother and father, complaining of extremely high fever for 4 days, with associated lethargy and malaise. His parents say he has not been himself since they returned from Disneyland Paris 5 days ago, and he seems 'off colour'. They deny vomiting, diarrhoea, dysuria or urinary frequency, sore throat or coryzal symptoms since onset of illness. He appears extremely tired and falls asleep during your consultation. When he is awake, he only verbalises yes and no answers and manages to point to his head and abdomen when you ask him if he is in any pain. He is normally fit and well and takes no regular medications.

Initial observations are recorded as HR 125, SpO$_2$ 97% on room air, RR 24, temperature 40°C (104.0°F), GCS 15/15. On examination, he appears warm peripherally, CRT <2 seconds centrally, moist mucous membranes. He is mildly tender across the entire abdomen, but the remainder of systemic examination is normal.

Upon further questioning, his parents disclose that prior to Disneyland, they had spent 3 weeks in Freetown, Sierra Leone, from where his parents originate. This is something they do frequently during the summer holidays. They inform you that they were in a closed compound, stayed only within the city, report use of mosquito nets and have no recollection of any bites. However, the child did not take any malaria prophylaxis or other travel vaccinations.

1. Which of the following is the best initial investigations and management for this patient?

    a. Bloods including FBC/U&Es/LFT/coagulation profile, empirical artesunate, IV crystalloid fluids, contact local paediatric critical care service for advice

    b. Bloods including FBC/U&Es/LFT/coagulation profile, thick and thin blood films, empirical quinine sulphate, refer to infectious diseases and paediatric teams for admission

    c. Bloods including FBC/U&Es/LFT/coagulation profile, thick and thin blood films, CBG, refer to infectious diseases and paediatric teams for admission

    d. Bloods including FBC/U&Es/LFT/coagulation profile, CBG, refer to paediatric team for admission

    e. Bloods including FBC/U&Es/LFT/coagulation profile, oral fluid challenge, refer to infectious diseases and paediatric teams for admission

DOI: 10.1201/9781003461456-33

The thin film is performed.

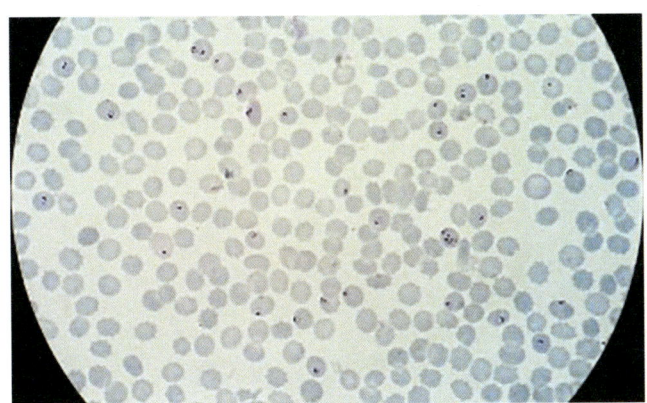

2. Which of the following organisms is seen in the image?

   a. *Plasmodium vivax*

   b. *Plasmodium malariae*

   c. *Trypanosoma brucei*

   d. *Plasmodium falciparum*

   e. *Trypanosoma cruzi*

The film is reported as having a parasitic load of 24%.

3. What would be the most appropriate initial pharmacological management for malaria in this child?

   a. Artemether/Lumefantrine (Riamet): 2 tablets PO @ 0, 8, 24, 36, 48 and 60 hours

   b. Quinine sulphate: 10 mg/kg (max 600 mg) PO TDS for 7 days

   c. Artemether/Lumefantrine (Riamet): 2 tablets PO TDS for 7 days

   d. Quinine dihydrochloride: 10 mg/kg IV TDS for 48 hours

   e. Artesunate: 2.4 mg/kg IV at 0, 12 and 24 hours, then OD

☑ 1c Bloods including FBC/U&Es/LFT/coagulation profile, thick and thin blood films, CBG, refer to infectious diseases and paediatric teams for admission

Any patient with fever who has recently travelled to a malaria endemic region should have a full complement of blood tests, including samples for thick and thin blood films. Depending on local procedures you may need to alert your laboratory that you are sending samples for malaria film so that they can review these quickly to give an initial parasite load, which can help guide initial management. A capillary blood glucose is specifically indicated in the prognostication of malaria in children. Though slightly tachycardic for his age, he appears well hydrated and is able to take oral fluids meaning there is no current indication for IV fluid resuscitation; however, a line should be placed. Empirical treatment is not recommended except in extreme circumstances where there is a strong clinical suspicion of severe disease where prompt laboratory confirmation is not possible. Both the infectious diseases and paediatric teams should be consulted as he is likely to require admission. Referral to the local paediatric critical care service is indicated in cases of severe malaria with organ dysfunction. Indications of severe disease include cardiovascular instability/shock, acute respiratory distress, jaundice, impaired consciousness, anaemia, acute kidney injury, disseminated intravascular coagulation and/or high parasitic load. This patient has no symptoms suggestive of severe disease; it is appropriate to manage locally at this stage.

☑ 2d *Plasmodium falciparum*

The gold standard diagnostic test for malaria is microscopic examination of the blood film specimen, stained with Giemsa stain to give the parasites a typical appearance. *Plasmodium falciparum*, which is the most common organism causing malaria in Africa, has a trophocyte phase that shows characteristic fine 'ring-shaped' parasites within the erythrocytes. In the provided film, you should appreciate the high density of infected erythrocytes, including doubly parasitised cells. If the trophozoites display double chromatin dots, then this is pathognomic for falciparum. *Plasmodium vivax* is the second most common cause of malaria worldwide but is more often seen in South-East Asia. It typically infects reticulocytes rather than mature erythrocytes. Its trophocyte phase is typically 'ameboid' with Schüffner's dots. *Plasmodium malariae* is typically seen in sub-Saharan Africa, but often causes less severe disease than *P. falciparum*. The trophocyte phase appears far darker (almost black) than *P. falciparum* on blood films and is typically 'band-' or 'sash-like' in structure. *P. malariae* may also be diagnosed by the 'rosette' form where merozoites line around the perimeter of the schizont with a highly pigmented centre. *Trypanosoma brucei* (African sleeping sickness) is an intracellular parasite transmitted by the tsetse fly; this parasite travels through the lymphatic system into the plasma travelling to the CNS but does not commonly infect erythrocytes. *Trypanosoma cruzi* causes Chagas disease. These are intracellular parasites transmitted by triatomine bugs in the Americas, but again do not tend to infect erythrocytes.

☑   3e Artesunate: 2.4 mg/kg IV at 0, 12 and 24 hours, then OD

Based on identifying the correct organism (*P. falciparum*) and the parasite count of an astonishing 24%, this patient should be treated as severe malarial infection. As well as prompt administration of drug therapy, you should strongly consider discussing with the local paediatric critical care service as he may need transfer to paediatric intensive care unit (ICU). IV artesunate is first-line therapy in severe infection and is given 12-hourly for three doses before switching to a once-daily regimen. If there is good response, the infectious diseases team may opt to switch to oral therapy following the first few doses of artesunate. IV quinine should only be used if IV artesunate is not immediately available. Once artesunate is available for administration, the patient should be switched immediately. Subsequent treatment of severe malaria should be guided by the infectious diseases team. Artemether/lumefantrine (Riamet) is an oral-only therapy that can be used first line in uncomplicated malaria, or to continue treatment following initial IV therapy. The dosing is weight-based and has a strict timing schedule which must be adhered to. Oral quinine is acceptable as initial management of uncomplicated malaria, but only if it has not been used for malaria prophylaxis. This patient was discussed with the paediatric critical care service but was felt suitable to continue management at his local hospital and did not require ICU admission. He was treated with IV artesunate for 2 days before switching to oral artemether/lumefantrine. After 3 days, the parasitic load was <0.1% and he was discharged home the following day.

KEY LEARNING POINTS

- History, history, history: information is key and the art of history-taking requires you to pick up on cues from the patient and relatives to tease out all of the relevant information.
- *Plasmodium falciparum* has distinctive features on blood film, including fine 'ring-shaped' trophozoites with double chromatin dots.
- IV artesunate is first line treatment in the management of severe malaria once diagnosis is confirmed, but IV quinine can be used if delay in obtaining artesunate.

CASE 34

Hyperlactataemia

A 72-year-old woman is brought into the emergency department (ED) by ambulance with significant generalised abdominal pain and an episode of syncope. You receive the patient directly in the resuscitation room.

Initial observations are recorded as HR 115, BP 95/47, SpO$_2$ 99% on 15L non-rebreathe mask, RR 28, temperature 36.5°C (97.7°F), GCS 15/15. On examination, she looks unwell. Her airway is patent, and chest is clear to auscultation. She is peripherally cool to the elbows with a thready radial pulse. Her abdomen is mildly distended and generally tender, but not peritonitic.

A venous blood gas (VBG) is performed, which reveals pH 7.121, pCO$_2$ 4.96, HCO$_3^-$ 11.7, BE –17.2, CBG 21.8, Lactate 12.3, Hb 126.

1. Regarding shock, which of the following statements is FALSE?

   a. Blood lactate is often elevated in all forms of shock, indicating the presence of tissue hypoxia

   b. The q-SOFA score is comprised of respiratory rate, mental status and blood pressure

   c. Shock is defined as a state of cellular and tissue hypoxia, where oxygen delivery is decreased relative to oxygen consumption

   d. A mean arterial pressure of <60 mmHg is required to 'diagnose' shock

   e. Class II haemorrhagic shock is associated with blood loss of 15–30% circulating volume

Following resuscitation, given the presentation you elect to perform an urgent CT abdomen & pelvis with contrast.

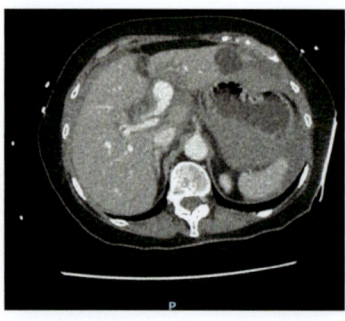

DOI: 10.1201/9781003461456-34

2. Which of the following is the correct CT conclusion?

    a. There is a large, irregular, soft tissue density within the rectum causing proximal bowel obstruction. There are multi-lobular hypodense lesions of the liver most likely representing metastatic disease

    b. There is a common hepatic artery aneurysm (HAA) with large volume ascites of increased density compatible with blood products suggestive of recent bleed from the site

    c. There is a thickened, inflamed segment of the sigmoid colon in keeping with acute diverticulitis. There is a large local collection containing fluid and gas, as well as small volume pneumoperitoneum

    d. No anatomical cause for the patient's symptoms is identified

    e. Liquefactive necrosis of the pancreatic parenchyma with high-attenuation fluid in the retroperitoneum and peri-pancreatic tissues. Findings are consistent with acute, necrotising pancreatitis

The metabolic status continues to improve following initial resuscitation, such that her lactate is now 6.6 and pH is 7.321.

Blood pressure remains 95/50 mmHg after 2.5 litres of intravenous crystalloid fluid.

3. Based on the CT findings above and current clinical parameters, which of these is the best ongoing management plan?

    a. Invasive monitoring (arterial & CVC line), 1g tranexamic acid IV, resuscitation with blood products, referral to interventional radiology, general surgery & intensive care unit (ICU)

    b. Invasive monitoring (arterial & CVC line), resuscitation with blood products and/or vasopressors, refer to infectious diseases team

    c. Invasive monitoring (arterial & CVC line), continue IV fluid resuscitation, broad-spectrum IV antibiotics such as cefuroxime & metronidazole

    d. Continue IV fluid resuscitation, broad-spectrum IV antibiotics such as cefuroxime & metronidazole, site NG tube, refer to general surgery

    e. Commence fixed rate insulin infusion 0.1 unit/kg/hour and refer to acute internal medicine team

☑ 1d A mean arterial pressure of <60 mmHg is required to 'diagnose' shock

Shock is often diagnosed when signs of hypoperfusion are associated with low or declining blood pressure. It may result from a number of disease processes, including pump failure (cardiogenic), loss of intravascular volume (hypovolaemic), failure of vaso-regulation (vasoplegic/distributive) or obstruction to blood flow (obstructive). At the cellular level, oxygen delivery becomes insufficient to meet oxygen demand for aerobic metabolism, meaning cells switch to anaerobic metabolism, which is seen biochemically as a raised lactate. Remember in anaerobic metabolism glucose is converted to 2 pyruvate molecules via glycolysis leading to net production of 2 ATP molecules. Pyruvate is then converted to lactate. The original Sequential Organ Failure Assessment (SOFA) score includes laboratory values, thus delaying diagnosis of shock via this method. The qSOFA uses three basic parameters that can be used in the pre-hospital setting and in the ED, assigning 1 point for hypotension (systolic BP ≤100 mmHg), tachypnoea (≥22 breaths per minute), or altered sensorium (GCS <15/15). Hypotension is not required in the diagnosis of shock; neurohumeral, sympathetic and parasympathetic mechanisms in shock can produce pulse rates and blood pressure that are normal, high or low.

☑ 2b There is a common hepatic artery aneurysm with large volume ascites of increased density compatible with blood products suggestive of recent bleed from the site

There is an aneurysm (~2–3 cm) arising from the common hepatic artery (best seen at 00m13s) with large volume ascites of increased density compatible with blood suggestive of recent bleed from the site. In addition, there is extensive fluid in the left subphrenic space, tracking along the paracolic gutters and pooling within the pelvis. There are multiple, bilobar, uniform hypodense lesions in the liver, which are likely to be simple cysts. There are multiple uncomplicated appearing sigmoid diverticula but no evidence of acute inflammation or perforation. In contrast, in active diverticulitis look for pericolic fat stranding, segmental bowel wall thickening or extravasation of gas and fluid into pelvis/peritoneum if perforated. There are normal appearances of the pancreas, distended and thin-walled gallbladder, adrenals and non-obstructed kidneys. Acute pancreatitis is usually associated with focal or diffuse parenchymal enlargement, changes in density due to oedema, indistinct pancreatic margins due to inflammation and retroperitoneal fat stranding, none of which are present on this scan.

☑ 3a Invasive monitoring (arterial & CVC line), 1 g tranexamic acid IV, resuscitation with blood products, referral to interventional radiology, general surgery & intensive care unit (ICU)

In spite of the initial improvement and based on the diagnosis of a ruptured HAA, it is clear that the patient requires urgent intervention to control the source of bleeding, which the interventional radiology (IR) team can provide. She remains haemodynamically unstable despite fluid resuscitation, requiring urgent transfusion of packed red cells plus additional products based on estimated blood loss and coagulation profile, along with continuous BP monitoring with an arterial line and/or vasopressors (i.e. she requires ICU level care). HAA is a rare disease with a prevalence of <0.5%, but with a high rupture rate of ~44%. The management of a leaking HAA, as is the case with any shock secondary to massive haemorrhage, is prompt resuscitation followed by urgent definitive management to stop bleeding. In this case, the first line, where possible, is hepatic artery embolisation and stenting by IR. Surgical intervention is generally indicated if the patient continues to deteriorate or if endovascular intervention fails.

Watch the IR angiogram clearly showing the size of the HAA.

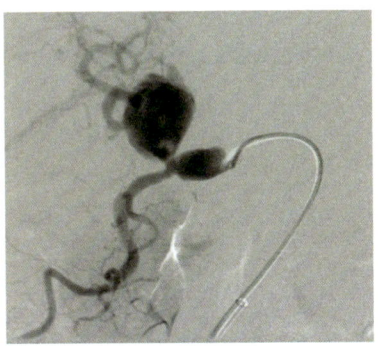 

KEY LEARNING POINTS

- Shock is a clinical syndrome characterised by inadequate blood flow to tissues resulting in cellular hypoxia, lactate production and a switch to anaerobic metabolism.
- Hepatic artery aneurysms are a rare entity overall but have a rate of spontaneous rupture of up to 44% and mortality of 80–100%.
- Treatment options for hepatic artery aneurysm rupture include open surgical procedures (ligation, aneurysmectomy with end-to-end anastomosis, aneurysmorrhaphy, bypass grafting) or endovascular techniques (catheter-directed coil embolisation, exclusion with a covered stent or flow diverting stents).

I can't stop vomiting

A 21-year-old man of African descent presents to the emergency department with a 3-day history of generalised abdominal pain after multiple episodes of vomiting. He most recently opened his bowels 5 days prior and had no previous history of constipation. On systems review, he notes mild burning chest pain and occasional difficulty breathing. He reports being well prior to this presentation and has no past medical history.

Initial observations are recorded as HR 90, BP 137/99, SpO$_2$ 100% on room air, RR 20, temperature 37.3°C (99.1°F). Cardiovascular exam is normal, and chest auscultation reveals normal vesicular breath sounds. The abdomen is soft but globally tender to palpation with no guarding.

As part of the work-up a chest radiograph is performed.

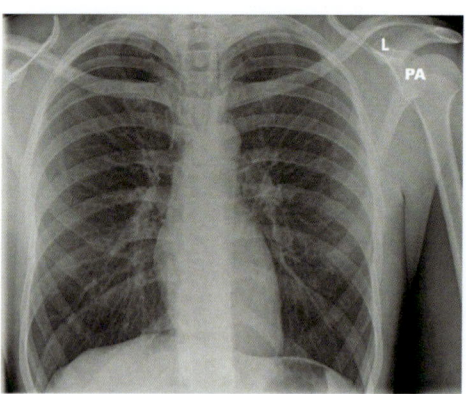

1. Which of the following is the best description of the findings of the chest radiograph?
   a. Pneumoperitoneum
   b. Apical pneumothorax
   c. Surgical emphysema
   d. Normal chest radiograph
   e. Left shoulder dislocation

DOI: 10.1201/9781003461456-35

You administer intravenous antiemetics and simple analgesia. There is no further vomiting whilst in the department, but the patient complains of persistent burning chest and upper abdominal pain.

You note the venous blood gas (VBG) revealed a Lactate of 3.1 and laboratory bloods reveal raised inflammatory markers with WCC 15.47, neutrophils 13.15, CRP 53.8 and renal function reveals creatinine 138 and eGFR 60.

2. Which of the following describes the next best management steps?

  a. Serial ECGs, continuous cardiac monitoring, send Troponin T, refer to acute internal medicine

  b. Pantoprazole 40 mg IV, broad-spectrum IV antibiotics, refer to acute internal medicine

  c. 1 L balanced crystalloid IV over 2 hours, repeat VBG after, aiming to discharge with outpatient follow-up if lactate and creatinine improves

  d. Amoxicillin 1 g + clarithromycin 500 mg + omeprazole 20 mg BD outpatient prescription, discharge for GP follow-up

  e. NBM, maintenance IV fluids with output chart, broad-spectrum IV antibiotics, refer to general surgeons

The following imaging is performed.

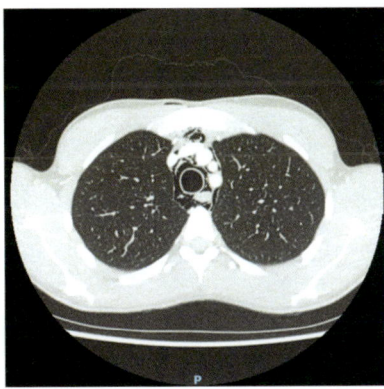 

3. Which of the following best describes the abnormality that is demonstrated?

  a. Pneumothorax

  b. Pericardial effusion

  c. Pneumomediastinum

  d. Pneumonia

  e. Pneumonitis

☑ 1c Surgical emphysema

The chest radiograph shows subtle gas within the superior mediastinum (look around the arch of the aorta on the left), consistent with pneumomediastinum and surgical emphysema evident in the supraclavicular regions best seen on the right. These findings are incredibly subtle, and you may find that it is easy to miss at first glance. This highlights the importance of a systemic method of reviewing chest radiographs to ensure all areas are assessed for abnormality. There are many methods, but one suggested technique is ABCDE approach for **A**irway (trachea, carina, bronchi, hilar), **B**reathing (lungs, pleura), **C**ardiac (heart, great vessels and their borders), **D**iaphragm (including costophrenic angles and under the diaphragm), **E**verything else (bones, soft tissues, artefacts including tubes/lines/implantable devices and review areas: lung apices, behind the heart, lung peripheries, hilar regions). Here the lungs and pleural spaces are clear and there is no apical pneumothorax which could account for the surgical emphysema. There is no air under the diaphragm suggesting pneumoperitoneum and the left shoulder joint appears normal.

☑ 2e NBM, maintenance IV fluids with output chart, broad-spectrum IV antibiotics, refer to general surgeons

The clinical history should help guide the answer here. The most important diagnosis to exclude with this history of torrential vomiting and burning chest pain along with the subtle chest radiograph changes suggestive of air entering the mediastinum and subcutaneous tissue is Boerhaave syndrome. Broad principles of management should include keeping the patient nil by mouth to prevent further contamination of the mediastinum, covering with broad-spectrum antibiotics to treat mediastinitis, and referring to the general surgeons who may elect to treat this conservatively if the leak is small or surgical repair of the oesophageal leak. Some centres may need to refer to specialist units where they have dedicated upper gastrointestinal surgeons who have more experience in surgical management. Prior to any intervention, definitive imaging to further assess location of injury and extend of contamination is required; in this case proceeding to CT chest with both IV and oral contrast will allow for full assessment. Mortality associated with Boerhaave syndrome is high at around 35% and so this should be treated as a true surgical emergency. Note that the renal function here could be normal for this man, as ethnicity and muscle mass can influence creatinine levels, but acute kidney injury is the more likely possibility secondary to dehydration from profuse vomiting.

☑ 3c Pneumomediastinum

The most striking abnormality here is the large volume pneumomediastinum seen on the lung window setting. You will note the 'black' air tracking through the neck soft tissue planes (surgical emphysema) and then tracking down into the chest and mediastinum.

To determine whether the air leak is from the trachea or oesophagus, both IV and oral contrast was given. This did not show any convincing evidence of oesophageal rupture, which would have been suggested by oesophageal wall thickening and oral contrast extravasation from the oesophagus, and so the leak was thought to have been caused by a small airway rupture whilst vomiting. This patient was managed conservatively. The subacute history and minimal physiological derangement also correspond with this cause of the pneumomediastinum compared to an oesophageal rupture. Oesophageal ruptures vary in severity, but the two main categories are superficial mucosal (Mallory–Weiss tear) and full-thickness ruptures. Full-thickness rupture allows leakage of stomach contents into the mediastinum and pleural cavity, triggering a severe inflammatory response that quickly deteriorates into physiological derangement, sepsis and a mortality rate of 35%.

KEY LEARNING POINTS

- A systematic approach to the interpretation of chest radiographs reduces the chances of missing subtle findings.
- A CT with both oral and IV contrast should be given to determine the site of leak in patients with pneumomediastinum.
- Patients should be managed as a true surgical emergency with covering antibiotics, parenteral analgesia, PPIs and prompt referral due to high mortality rates.

In a place called vertigo

A 47-year-old woman presents to the emergency department after waking with a right-sided headache and right neck pain. The pain improves with oral analgesia, but returns a few hours later associated with dizziness, with nausea but no vomiting. She reports her symptoms are worse when she opens her eyes. She denies any recent illness or trauma. She suffers with frequent migraines. She smokes around 15–20 cigarettes per day and describes feeling extremely stressed due to the recent bereavement of her partner.

Initial observations are recorded as HR 75, BP 116/56, SpO_2 99% on room air, RR 17, temperature 36.8°C (98.2°F). Examination is difficult due to extreme symptoms on eye opening. Head impulse, nystagmus, test of skew (HINTS) examination reveals no corrective saccade on head impulse with 2 beats of horizontal nystagmus to the right. The cranial nerve examination that can be assessed is normal. You cannot assess gait as the patient cannot stand due to symptoms, but the remainder of the peripheral nerve examination is grossly normal.

A venous blood gas (VBG) has been obtained and you note pH 7.456, Lactate 4.5, CBG 6.3.

Bloods are drawn including FBC, U&Es, CRP and coagulation profile.

1. Which of the following would you include in your initial management plan for this patient?
    a. Prochlorperazine 12.5 mg IM and request urgent CT head with angiogram
    b. Prochlorperazine 12.5 mg IM and perform an Epley manoeuvre
    c. Sumatriptan 20 mg intranasally and observe
    d. Non-contrast CT head and admit for lumbar puncture if negative
    e. Sumatriptan 6 mg SC and high-flow oxygen via a tight-fitting mask for 30 minutes

DOI: 10.1201/9781003461456-36

The patient is admitted due to her symptoms and has an MRI as part of her inpatient journey.

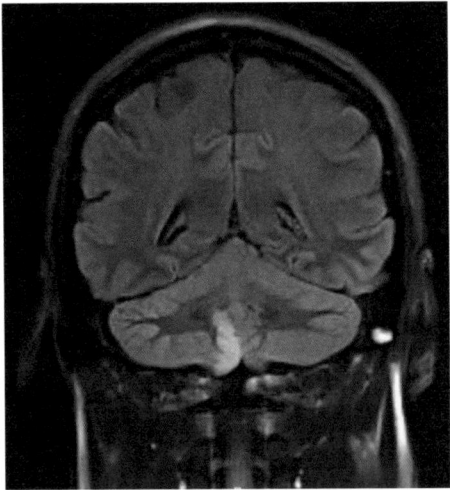

2. Which of the following is the best description of what is shown in the image?

   a. Multiple white matter lesions suggesting acute demyelinating disease

   b. Small volume subarachnoid bleed in keeping with a sentinel bleed from a cerebral aneurysm

   c. Lateral medullary infarct associated with Wallenberg syndrome

   d. White matter hyperintensities in keeping with chronic migraines

   e. Acute infarcts in the region of the posterior inferior communicating artery

3. Which of the following would make you most suspicious of a posterior circulation stroke as opposed to a migraine?

   a. Corrective saccade on head impulse test on HINTS examination

   b. Neck pain with absence of vertigo

   c. Absence of aura

   d. Sports exercise preceding the onset of symptoms

   e. Improvement of headache after analgesia

☑ 1a Prochlorperazine 12.5 mg IM and request urgent CT head with angiogram

The correct answer is to administer an antiemetic such as prochlorperazine and request CT head with angiogram. The clinical picture is slightly tricky in this case. At first you may think this could be a migraine – known history, prior 'headache' and limited vomiting – but the key discriminator here is the vertiginous symptoms. Our next question is whether this is due to a peripheral cause (for example, benign paroxysmal positional vertigo [BPPV], vestibular neuritis, Ménière's disease) or a central cause for example, posterior circulation stroke, multiple sclerosis or posterior fossa tumour. The HINTS examination can help us work this out but should only be used if there is persistent vertigo over hours or days, nystagmus and normal neurological examination. A central cause is suggested by negative head impulse (absence of corrective saccade), bidrectional nystagmus or abnormal movement on test of skew. In this case it is abnormal, suggesting a central lesion and so the best and safest answer is to perform a CT head with angiogram. The other answers are treatments for: BPPV (prochlorperazine & Epley manoeuvre), migraine (sumatriptan 20 mg IN), SAH with sentinel bleed (non-contrast CT and lumbar puncture) and cluster headache (sumatriptan 6 mg SC and high-flow oxygen therapy).

☑ 2e Acute infarcts in the region of the posterior inferior communicating artery

This a coronally reformatted, T2-weighted, MRI scan of the brain with fat suppression. The key abnormalities are the hyperdense (white lesions) in the right cerebellum. This confirms an acute posterior inferior cerebellar artery (PICA) infarct. This patient did in fact have a CT head with angiogram prior to the MRI, but the acute infarct was not visualised. However, there was suggestion of a small area of possible dissection near the vertebral artery. This was subsequently shown to be a congenitally narrow segment with atheroma on the MRI. The learning point is that CT remains the first line investigation as it will reveal large bleeds, tumours, large infarcts and cerebromalacia. However, due to its poor sensitivity in identification of strokes in the posterior circulation, particularly the posterior fossa structures, in the presence of ongoing symptoms the patient should receive input from neurology and/or stroke specialist teams and additional neuroimaging with MRI.

☑ 3d Sports exercise preceding the onset of symptoms

In terms of the options, that which would be most suspicious of a posterior circulation stroke is sports exercise preceding the onset of symptoms. This is because traumatic dissection of the vertebral artery is one of the most common causes of posterior stroke in younger patients. Though this patient did not have any history of trauma, if she had done the suspicion of stroke would have been even higher. Considering the alternative options, abnormal head impulse (i.e. absence of corrective saccade) indicates a central lesion as opposed to peripheral cause of vertigo, neck pain if associated with symptoms suspicious of posterior stroke may be due to vertebral artery dissection, which can lead to stroke, absence of aura does not preclude a headache being due to migraine but the other symptoms in this case point you away from migraine here, and improvement in headache with analgesia should not reassure you given the atypical symptoms and signs in this patient. Remember there are a number of risk factors for stroke including hypertension, diabetes mellitus, ischaemic heart disease, hypercholesterolaemia, smoking and family history – from the provided history, we know that the patient is a smoker and it transpires that she also had a cousin who had a significant stroke in their 40s.

KEY LEARNING POINTS

- A HINTS examination can be helpful in discriminating between central and peripheral causes of vertigo but needs the patient to be acutely symptomatic.
- MRI is the preferred modality over CT in detecting posterior fossa ischaemic events. However, CT with angiogram of the cerebral vessels still remains the first line investigation in acute presentations.
- Apart from the common risk factors of stroke, vertebral artery dissection is an important cause of posterior circulation stroke, especially in young patients.

Just constipation?

A 61-year-old female presents with a 1-week history of nausea and vomiting. She has only opened her bowels once in this time and has had progressively increasing abdominal pain and distention. She has recently completed her third cycle of chemotherapy for a tubo-ovarian malignancy.

Observations are all within normal limits. On examination, she is slightly cool peripherally with a central capillary refill time of 2 seconds; the abdomen is moderately distended with generalised tenderness and bowel sounds are high pitched.

Initial venous blood gas (VBG) is unremarkable with a Lactate of 2.0.

A CT abdomen & pelvis with contrast is performed.

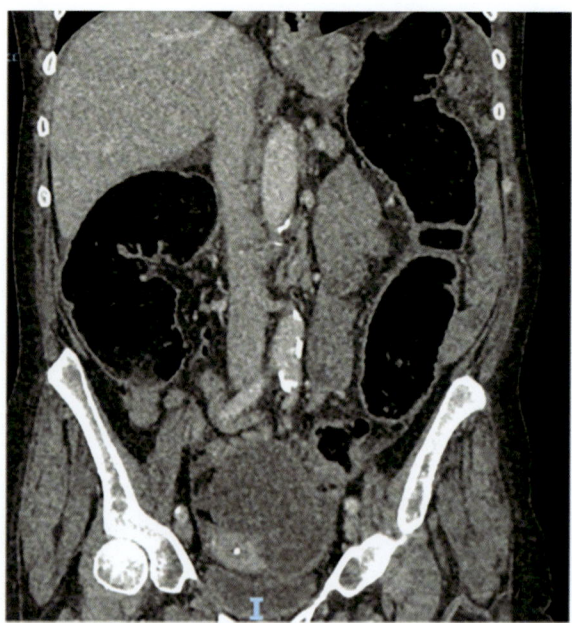

DOI: 10.1201/9781003461456-37

1. What are the units used to describe the radiograph densities in the body associated with CT?
   a. Hounsford units
   b. Houston units
   c. Godfrey units
   d. Holmbrey units
   e. Hounsfield units

2. With which of the following diagnoses is the displayed imaging consistent?
   a. Ovarian torsion
   b. Small bowel obstruction
   c. Large bowel obstruction
   d. Infected pelvic collection
   e. Faecal impaction

You review the laboratory results and note a WCC of 14 (neuts 12), CRP 2. The remaining full blood count, renal function and electrolytes are all within normal limits.

3. Based on the blood results and CT findings, what is your initial management plan?
   a. Draw blood cultures, administer broad-spectrum IV antibiotics
   b. Insert wide-bore NG tube, NBM, IV fluid replacement
   c. Perform high vaginal swabs and administer oral antibiotics
   d. Administer phosphate enema +/– oral laxatives and review
   e. Arrange an urgent transvaginal ultrasound scan

☑ 1e Hounsfield units

CT is based on the principle that density of tissues is measured from calculating the attenuation coefficient. This allows the density of the body to be reconstructed into a 2D section perpendicular to the axis of the detector. The detectors measure the transmission of a thin beam of radiographs through a section of the body from multiple different angles, which provides information of depth and therefore the third dimension. Hounsfield units (HU) are a dimensionless unit used in CT. They are obtained from a linear transformation of the measured attenuation coefficients, which are a measure of the degree of penetration of an incident energy beam by a material. The linear transformation is based on the assigned densities at standard temperature and pressure (STP) of air (radiodensity at STP = −1000 HU) and pure water (radiodensity at STP = 0 HU). The scale runs from −1000 HU for air to around +2000 HU for very dense bone (for example, cochlea) and over +3000 HU for metals. The units are named after the Nobel prize winner and inventor of CT, Sir Godfrey Hounsfield.

☑ 2c Large bowel obstruction

The displayed coronal image shows distention of both the ascending and descending colon due to an obstruction in the region of the sigmoid colon. The small bowel, however, is not distended as you can see segments of collapsed small bowel either side of the descending colon as well as a small portion of the terminal ileum, which is also collapsed; this is due to a competent ileocecal valve that prevents decompression of the distended colon. CT is the most widely used imaging modality for assessing bowel obstruction as it is more sensitive than plain films and, as well as confirming the diagnosis, in most cases it is able to identify the cause. Within this scan you can also identify a septated cystic lesion within the pelvis, in keeping with the patient's known malignancy. Features of ovarian torsion on CT include an enlarged ovary; an ovary that may be shifted to the midline or uterus displaced to the involved side, and fat stranding in the adnexa; however, ultrasound is often the first line imaging modality. A pelvic fluid collection would usually be seen as a relatively low attenuating central component with capsular ring enhancement with contrast and surrounding inflammatory changes, (for example, fat stranding).

☑ 3b Insert wide-bore NG tube, NBM, IV fluid replacement

The initial management for bowel obstruction is often referred to as 'drip and suck', referring to IV fluid maintenance +/− resuscitation of any fluid and electrolyte losses, and insertion of an NG tube that is left on free drainage. The majority of patients will also require a urinary catheter to assist strict fluid balance monitoring. Analgesia and antiemetics are also an important aspect of management. While this patient's WCC and neutrophils are raised, this is likely a mild inflammatory response. Clinically there are no features of sepsis, strangulation or peritonism. Therefore, blood cultures and antibiotics are not required at this stage. However, it may be prudent to administer broad-spectrum antibiotics should clinicals signs of sepsis exist according to local microbiology guidelines for example, cefuroxime + metronidazole. Given the history it would be worthwhile to involve both general surgery and oncology teams to establish her ongoing management. Based on where you are working, oncology teams may have a lot of experience looking after patients with malignant bowel obstruction. However, in other hospitals you will find the general surgery team managing the patients with oncology input. If there is no sign of ischaemia or perforation, initial management is most often conservative. In cases of small bowel obstruction, water soluble contrast study can be performed with an abdominal radiograph 6 hours after ingestion of oral contrast to see if there is resolution or ongoing obstruction. Gastrografin, which is often used in this setting, may also have therapeutic effects as it is thought to have an osmotic effect on bowel wall oedema. Surgical management (laparotomy) is indicated for bowel ischaemia, closed loop obstruction, reversible surgical causes (for example, strangulated hernia or obstructing tumour) or if patients fail to improve with conservative measures.

KEY LEARNING POINTS

- Hounsfield units are used in CT scans to measure structure density with metals being most dense (+3000), bone being intermediate (+2000) and air being least dense (−1000).
- Axial imaging such as CT is the preferred imaging modality as it may reveal the cause of bowel obstruction as well as the level of obstruction and transition points but it incurs a significant radiation dose and this should be considered.
- Bowel obstruction in patients with cancer may need multidisciplinary input from oncological, general surgical and radiology teams to get best outcomes. A conservative approach with IV rehydration, bowel decompression with an NG tube and fluid output monitoring is still the mainstay of initial treatment.

CASE 38

Loss of vision after an overdose

A 60-year-old man presents 5 days after an intentional mixed overdose of his own pre-scription bisoprolol, losartan and clopidogrel. In total, he believes he took a total of 80 tablets alongside five beers with suicidal intent. He did not seek medical attention, but awoke 24 hours later with altered vision and has since been bumping into objects whilst walking. On further questioning he also reports that 3 months previously he was hit by a car at <20 mph as a pedestrian and sustained a head injury but did not present to the emergency department. Since this time, he has noticed intermittent dizziness, feeling clumsy and loss of coordination.

Past medical history includes hypertension, previous coronary artery bypass graft, type 2 diabetes mellitus, hypercholesterolaemia, hepatic steatosis, chronic kidney disease stage 3 and alcohol excess (approximately 40 units per day).

Initial observations are recorded as HR 84, BP 188/88, SpO_2 98% on room air, RR 18, temperature 36.4°C (97.5°F), GCS 15/15.

1. Which of the following options would NOT be included in your differentials at this stage?

   a. Wernicke's encephalopathy

   b. Bisoprolol toxicity

   c. Stroke

   d. Angiotensin-II receptor antagonist toxicity

   e. Subdural haematoma

You perform a focused neurological examination which reveals no facial droop or ptosis but pronounced dysdiadochokinesia on the left, a broad-based ataxic gait and an inability to heel-toe walk. On assessment of the visual system, the patient appears to display a left homonymous hemianopia; you cannot discern if there is macular sparing clinically. Direct fundoscopy and pupillary reflexes are grossly normal. Visual acuity is problematic due to patient compliance.

2. Which imaging modality is the single best option to confirm the suspected diagnosis?

   a. CT venogram

   b. Air contrast echocardiogram

   c. Non-contrast CT head

   d. CT head & CT angiogram stroke protocol

   e. MRI & MRA head

DOI: 10.1201/9781003461456-38

A non-contrast CT head is performed, and you review the images.

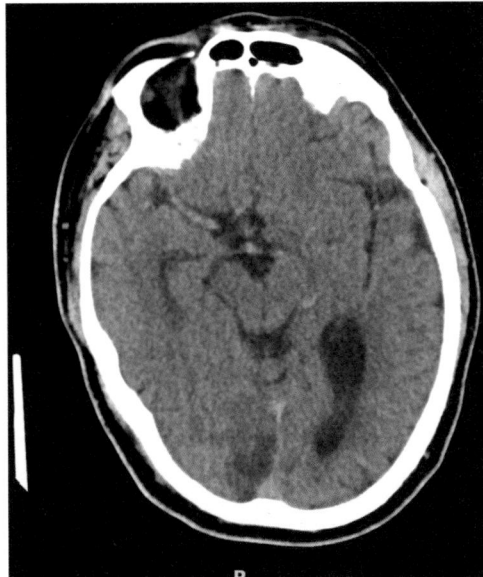

3. Which of the following reports is most likely to correspond to the findings seen?

  a. There is an area of hypodensity affecting the right occipital region cortical and subcortical in location and is likely to represent an established infarct; MRI is recommended for further delineation

  b. There is an area of hypodensity affecting the right occipital region cortical and subcortical in location and is likely to represent a space-occupying lesion; further evaluation with contrast is recommended

  c. There is an area of hypodensity affecting the right occipital region, which may represent a chronic bleed (is there a history of trauma?)

  d. There is unchanged background small vessel disease; no acute abnormality detected on this scan; no cause for patient's symptoms identified

  e. There are widened lateral ventricles and periventricular hypodensity, with dilation of the Sylvian fissure; clinical correlation is recommended

☑ 1b Bisoprolol toxicity

All options should be considered as potential differential diagnoses at this stage, except for beta-blocker toxicity. The patient is at risk of thiamine deficiency due to his excessive alcohol intake; the classic triad of Wernicke's encephalopathy is ataxia, impaired vision and confusion, though only 10% of patients have all three features. A history of head injury and neurology should always also prompt you to consider traumatic injury, for example subdural haematoma. Note that if present in this case, it would likely be chronic. Visual disturbance, loss of coordination and dizziness should also make you consider a potential stroke, especially in a patient with multiple risk factors, though a full neurological examination is required. Losartan is an angiotensin-II receptor antagonist, which in overdose can cause dizziness and electrolyte disturbances, therefore should be considered. However, the most prominent effect is a profound hypotension and due to peak plasma concentration at 1–4 hours and half-life of approximately 1.5–9 hours, this is a less likely option. Beta-blocker toxicity features are relative to type of drug and amount taken, and include bradycardia, hypotension, AV block, hypoglycaemia, seizures and coma. Peak plasma concentrations of bisoprolol are reached between 1 and 3 hours after ingestion. Given the delayed presentation and absence of these features, this is the least likely option.

☑ 2e MRI & MRA head

The concern here, based on the collection of above symptoms, is posterior circulation infarction, which corresponds to any infarction within the vertebrobasilar vascular territory (brainstem, cerebellum, midbrain, thalami and areas of the temporal and occipital lobes). They account for 20% of ischaemic strokes. Clinical syndromes correspond to site of blood flow occlusion; common symptoms and signs include vertigo, dysarthria, dysphagia, ataxia, gaze palsy or diplopia and/or visual field deficits. Less than 1% of patients present with one symptom. CT is the main brain imaging modality in the hyperacute stroke setting with the goals to exclude intracranial haemorrhage (which excludes thrombolysis), assess for features of early ischaemia and exclude stroke mimics such as a space occupying lesion. However, CT has a known limited sensitivity to assess posterior circulation strokes, especially posterior fossa structures. MRI is much more sensitive. CT is generally first line, but if high clinical suspicion and negative CT, proceeding to MRI is strongly recommended.

☑ 3a There is an area of hypodensity affecting the right occipital region cortical and subcortical in location and is likely to represent an established infarct; MRI is recommended for further delineation

The CT shows an area of hypodensity in the right occipital region that is cortical and subcortical in region. This is highly suggestive of an established infarction (cell death attributable to ischaemia). This is likely due to a profound hypotension following angiotensin-II receptor antagonist and beta-blocker overdose. Given that this patient presented 5 days after the suspected insult, this would class the stroke as acute (24 hours to 1 week). At this stage there is marked hypoattenuation with parenchymal swelling, which can result in mass effect and secondary infarcts. The CT report also comments on background small vessel disease, which is seen as diffuse non-enhancing white matter hypodensities. The displayed CT does not have the typical appearance of a chronic subdural haematoma, which would be seen as a hypodense crescentic or biconvex shape. Occasionally, the periphery may calcify showing a hyperdense area, and 75–85% of chronic subdurals are bilateral. Widened ventricles, periventricular hypodensities and dilation of the Sylvian fissure may be seen in normal pressure hydrocephalus, though again MRI is a superior imaging modality to identify this, especially with use of CSF flow cytometry.

KEY LEARNING POINTS

- Patients may present with end-organ effects, particularly after a delayed presentation post-intentional overdose.
- Review each medication individually and clinically correlate to the symptoms presented.
- MRI is superior to CT in imaging the posterior fossa, but CT still remains the first-line investigation in most emergency departments and hyperacute stroke units.

Lower abdominal distension

A 54-year-old woman presents to the emergency department (ED) with a week's history of progressively worsening lower abdominal pain and distension, which is worse in the left lower quadrant. The pain is described as constant but exacerbated by movement. She tells you she is nauseous but has not vomited. Bowels were last opened 5 days ago, and she is not passing flatus. She has not noticed any weight loss. Past medical history includes type 2 diabetes mellitus and chronic lower back pain. She has no surgical history.

Initial observations are recorded as HR 81, BP 114/59, SpO$_2$ 96% on room air, RR 24, temperature 37.1°C (98.8°F). On examination her lower abdomen appears distended and is tender, especially in the lower half. Guarding and rebound tenderness are present in the left iliac fossa. There are no palpable hernias. Bowel sounds are absent. Digital rectal examination reveals an empty rectum.

A CT abdomen & pelvis is arranged after a negative urinary pregnancy test.

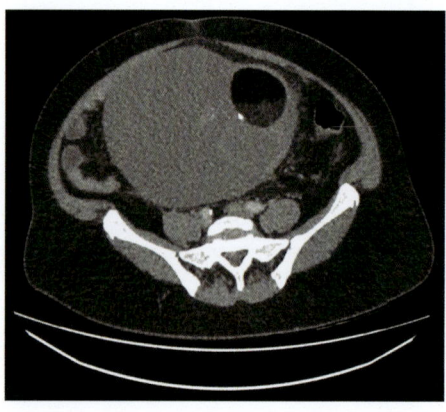 

1. Based on the findings, which of the following is the most likely diagnosis?

   a. Sigmoid obstruction due to tumour

   b. Perforated diverticulitis with abscess formation

   c. Ovarian torsion due to ovarian cyst

   d. Sigmoid volvulus

   e. Ovarian torsion due to cystic teratoma

DOI: 10.1201/9781003461456-39

You review the patient's previous imaging and note a subtle abnormality on a pelvis radiograph.

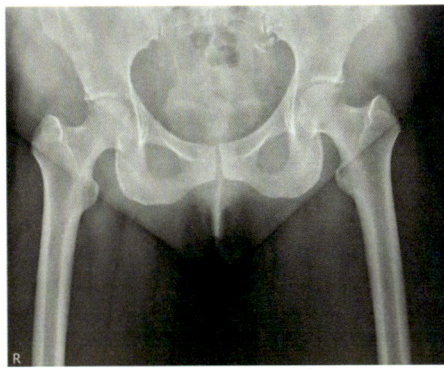

2. Which of the following is the best description of the observed abnormality?

   a. There is a soft tissue opacity in the pelvis above the pubic symphysis suggestive of multiple calcified fibroids

   b. Incidental mineralised object projected below the left SI joint, which appears to be surrounded by a high-density rounded focus measuring 9 cm across

   c. There is a lytic lesion in the sacral ala consistent with a metastatic lesion; clinical correlation is advised

   d. There is a step in the symphysis pubis suggestive of symphysis pubis dysfunction (does this patient have pain on walking or standing?)

   e. The bowel gas pattern appears to be abnormal near the rectum; clinical correlation is advised with a surgical opinion

3. Which cell types are thought to be implicated in the origin of pathological finding on the CT above?

   a. Endoderm, ectoderm and mesoderm

   b. Ectoderm only

   c. Mesoderm only

   d. Mitochondria and ectoderm

   e. Zona pellucida and mesoderm

☑ 1e Ovarian torsion due to cystic teratoma

The prominent abnormality on the CT is a large cystic lesion within the inferior abdomen and pelvis, appearing to arise from the left adnexa. A lesion this size with heterogeneity should point you towards a cystic teratoma, also called a 'dermoid cyst', rather than a simple ovarian cyst. Perilesional fat stranding, free fluid and twisted appearance of left broad ligament is suggestive of torsion. Although there appears to be a fluid level, there are no dilated bowel loops suggestive of bowel obstruction. Fat stranding and small amounts of free fluid may make you consider diverticulitis, but the lesion can be seen separate to the sigmoid colon. This woman was reviewed by general surgical and gynaecology teams and taken as an emergency case to theatre. Findings were of a large left-sided cyst with three rotations of the tube and ovary. Open left salpingectomy and oophorectomy was performed without complication, and she recovered well post-operatively.

☑ 2b Incidental mineralised object projected below the left SI joint, which appears to be surrounded by a high-density rounded focus measuring 9 cm across

Plain radiographs can identify calcific and tooth components present within mature cystic teratomas, and this can be seen as a lesion just below the left SIJ sitting in a rounded soft tissue mass. All of the other answers are incorrect: the apparent 'step' in symphysis pubis is due to a rotated film, the bowel gas shadowing is normal and there is no suggestion of lytic lesion in the sacral ala, and lastly the rounded soft tissue opacity in the pelvis represents the bladder and not a uterus with calcified fibroids. Ultrasound is the preferred imaging modality for ovarian cysts as although CT has high sensitivity, it is not routinely recommended in uncomplicated cysts due to ionising radiation. However, in the ED, CT is used to exclude other abdominal and pelvic pathologies particularly when there is no known history of ovarian cyst. Sonographic features of mature cystic teratomas can include echogenic mass with posterior sound attenuation due to sebaceous material within the cavity, presence of fluid levels, shadowing calcific or dental components and multiple thin echogenic bands in the cavity caused by hair.

☑ 3a Endoderm, ectoderm and mesoderm

A mature cystic teratoma is the most common of the three types of ovarian teratomas. It is a type of germ cell tumour (a tumour that begins in the cells that give rise to sperm or eggs). Histologically it includes at least two well-differentiated, mature germ cell layers (ectoderm, mesoderm, endoderm). The ectoderm and mesoderm are the most commonly seen germ cell layers in the tumour wall; therefore, mature tissues of the skin and hair (from the ectoderm) and fat and muscle (from the mesoderm) usually make up the composition of a mature cystic teratoma. Though they have similar imaging appearances, a dermoid cyst is composed of only dermal and epidermal elements, which are ectodermal in origin. It is still not completely understood how these develop but the most accepted theory is the parthenogenetic activation of oocytes (i.e. embryonic development without the male gamete) – the fact that the 46 XX karyotype is found in almost all mature teratomas strengthens this theory. Mature cystic teratomas account for around 15% of all ovarian neoplasms and tend to be identified in younger women around the age of 30 years. They are bilateral in 10–15% of cases.

KEY LEARNING POINTS

- Large cystic teratomas can mimic an acute surgical abdomen.
- Mature cystic teratomas can exist for years with little or few symptoms until they cause mass effect such as torsion, compression of surrounding structures or bowel obstruction.
- Plain radiograph may suggest their presence with calcific densities (teeth, calcified components) surrounded by a subtle soft tissue mass.

Message in a bottle

A 26-year-old man presents to the emergency department (ED) with 4 weeks of left-sided pleuritic chest pain radiating to the left shoulder, 2 weeks of dry cough and in the past week has been feeling feverish and short of breath on exertion. He uses cocaine recreationally once or twice a week and smokes 15 cigarettes per day with occasional cannabis use.

Initial observations are recorded as HR 101, BP 134/64, SpO_2 99% on room air, RR 16, temperature 37.7°C (99.9°F). You note clubbed fingernails. The remainder of the cardio-vascular and respiratory examination appear to be unremarkable.

The initial ECG is shown.

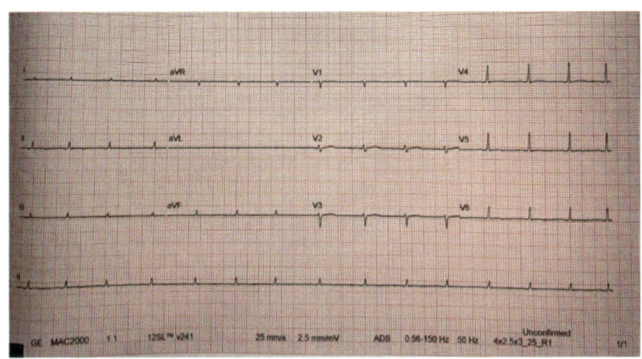 

1. What finding does this ECG suggest on first inspection?

   a. Delta waves

   b. Electrical alternans

   c. T-wave inversion

   d. Pathological Q waves

   e. Low voltage QRS

DOI: 10.1201/9781003461456-40

You note an abnormality on his chest radiograph.

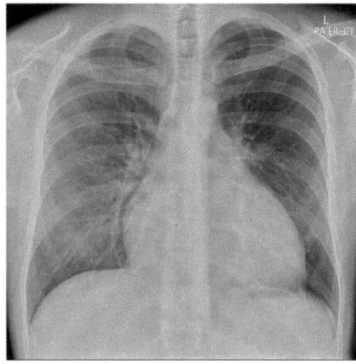 

2. Which single investigation available in the ED could most quickly confirm your suspected clinical diagnosis?

   a. CT pulmonary angiogram

   b. Point-of-care ultrasound (POCUS) echocardiogram

   c. High-resolution CT chest with contrast

   d. No further investigation required

   e. Cardiac MRI

You review the laboratory blood results and note CRP 135 and D-dimer 4300.

Observations remain as per booking in.

A CT pulmonary angiogram (CTPA) is performed due to the elevated D-dimer.

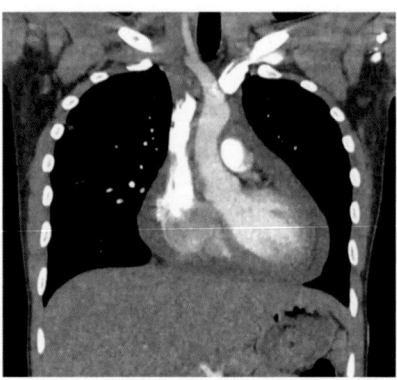 

3. What would you do next based on the CTPA and blood results?

  a. Weigh patient, administer treatment dose low molecular weight heparin, discharge with follow-up in the acute internal medicine hot clinic

  b. Advise to stop smoking, send sputum for acid-fast bacillus screen, discharge with referral to outpatient TB clinic

  c. Refer to the acute internal medicine team for a formal echocardiogram, viral screen, cardiology and infectious disease consults

  d. Prescribe oral colchicine 0.5 mg BD and co-amoxiclav 625 mg TDS for 7 days, discharge with follow-up in the acute internal medicine hot clinic

  e. Arrange for time-critical transfer to local cardiothoracic centre for endovascular aneurysm (EVAR) repair

☑ 1e Low voltage QRS

This ECG shows sinus tachycardia (rate 101) with apparent 'low voltage' QRS complexes. However, if you look carefully, you will note that there is a non-standard ECG setting of 2.5 mm/mV rather than the normal 10 mm/mV. There are P waves visible in V5 and V6 but they are generally hard to see across the recording due to the low amplitude complexes. There is flattening of the T waves but no convincing T-wave inversion. The delta wave is a slurred upstroke in the QRS complex, which relates to pre-excitation of the ventricles; it is often associated with shortening of the PR interval and seen in Wolff–Parkinson–White syndrome. Electrical alternans is when consecutive, normally conducted QRS complexes alternate in height due to the heart 'swinging' anteriorly and posteriorly within a large fluid-filled pericardium; there is no convincing evidence of this here. Electrical alternans is a specific (but insensitive) ECG finding of large pericardial effusion with tamponade.

☑ 2b Point-of-care ultrasound (POCUS) echocardiogram

This chest radiograph shows cardiomegaly (cardiac shadow >50% thoracic width) with a 'globe-shaped' heart; this is sometimes referred to as the 'water-bottle sign'. There is also sharp definition of the cardiac border, and one could argue a slight change in lucency at the inferior aspect of the apex. These findings, alongside the history and ECG should make you think about pericardial effusion. A POCUS echocardiogram is the quickest way to assess for pericardial fluid and ultrasound evidence of impending tamponade which includes right atrial systolic collapse, right ventricular diastolic collapse and distended inferior vena cava with no respiratory variation. An anechoic separation of pericardial layers can be identified on transthoracic echocardiogram (TTE) when pericardial fluid is >50 mL.

☑ 3c Refer to the acute internal medical team for a formal echocardiogram, viral screen, cardiology and infectious disease consults

The coronal reconstruction CTPA shows a large pericardial effusion. There is no pulmonary embolus (PE) and so treatment dose low molecular weight heparin is incorrect. Pericardial effusions are commonly associated with pericarditis; colchicine is recommended alongside NSAIDs for pericarditis but given the size of the effusion and uncertain aetiology this patient is unsafe for discharge at this stage and requires further investigation. There are multiple causes of pericardial effusion, including idiopathic, infectious (including viral, bacterial, TB), autoimmune (including systemic lupus erythematous, rheumatoid arthritis, ankylosing spondylitis), sarcoidosis, hypothyroidism, post-radiotherapy or cardiac surgery and drug induced (including hydralazine, isoniazid, minoxidil, phenytoin). Blood cultures, autoantibodies, viral serology, thyroid function tests, as well as a formal echocardiogram should be considered. Pericardiocentesis is indicated when there are either radiological (echocardiography) or clinical signs of tamponade (for example, hypotension, tachycardia). A surgical approach may be needed for chronic or loculated effusions. After investigation, this patient's effusion was found to be due to Epstein–Barr virus associated pericarditis. He was discharged on oral naproxen and colchicine with repeat outpatient echocardiogram, which showed full resolution of the effusion.

KEY LEARNING POINTS

- Always remember to perform basic setting checks (speed of paper, deflection settings) when interpreting ECGs, especially in the presence of abnormal findings.
- Point-of-care echocardiography is a useful adjunct in the breathless patient and can diagnose significant pericardial effusions and allow assessment of RV and LV function.
- In patients with risk factors for atypical infection such as drug misuse, a short admission provides a safe mechanism to get relevant tests performed in a timely manner.

My arm doesn't feel right

A 58-year-old man presents to the emergency department (ED) after a mechanical fall at home in his bathroom onto his right side hitting a glass shower screen. He described his right arm as 'limp and dead', hanging by his side after he stood up from the fall. He had no loss of consciousness or other red flag symptoms. He is usually fit and well and takes anti-retroviral medication for well controlled HIV.

On examination, he looks uncomfortable but on inspection there is no deformity of the shoulder or the arm. He is tender over the humeral shaft and movement is limited due to pain.

Radiographs of the shoulder are requested.

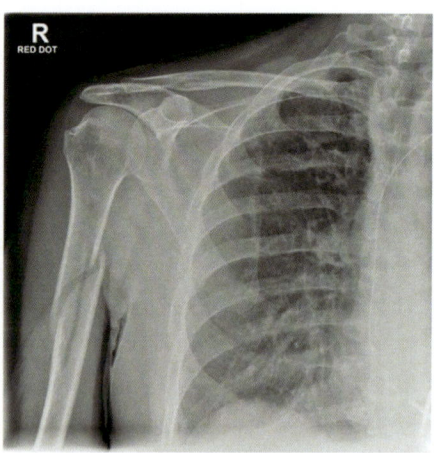 

1. With the pattern of injury shown in the radiograph, which anatomical structure is most at risk of damage?
   a. Median nerve
   b. Radial nerve
   c. Ulnar nerve
   d. Axillary nerve
   e. Musculocutaneous nerve

DOI: 10.1201/9781003461456-41

2. Which of the following best describes the function of the aforementioned structure?

    a. Motor innervation to majority of small hand muscles and sensation to the little and medial half of ring finger

    b. Main nerve to the forearm, supplying flexors of the wrist and sensation to majority of the volar aspect of the palm

    c. Motor innervation to three muscles and sensation to the regimental badge area

    d. Motor innervation to extensors of the forearm and sensory innervation to back of hand including the first web space

    e. Motor innervation to coracobrachialis, brachialis and biceps brachii and sensory innervation to lateral forearm

3. How would you manage a patient with this fracture pattern?

    a. Apply broad arm sling, discharge with referral to fracture clinic

    b. Apply collar & cuff, discharge with referral to fracture clinic

    c. Physiotherapy assessment and if passes, discharge with no follow-up

    d. Apply U-slab or humeral brace, referral to orthopaedics

    e. Request CT upper arm to assist operative planning, referral to orthopaedics

☑ 1b Radial nerve

The radial nerve runs from behind the axillary artery and dives down to enter the lower triangular space to reach the radial sulcus (also termed 'spiral groove') of the back of the humerus, where it is vulnerable to damage with spiral fractures of the humeral shaft as is seen in the radiograph. The median nerve enters the arm from the axilla at the inferior margin of the teres major and passes vertically down, lateral to the brachial artery before crossing anteriorly to run medially to the artery. The ulnar nerve, in comparison, descends medial to the brachial artery until the insertion point of the coracobrachialis; it then pierces the medial intermuscular septum and enters the posterior compartment of the arm. It runs at the posteromedial aspect of the humerus, passing behind the medial epicondyle. The axillary nerve passes down the lower border of the subscapularis before winding anterior to posterior around the surgical neck of the humerus.

☑ 2d Motor innervation to extensors of the forearm and sensory innervation to back of hand including the first web space

The radial nerve provides motor innervation to the dorsal arm muscles and extrinsic extensors of the wrists and hands; it provides cutaneous sensory innervation to most of the back of the hand, except the little finger and medial half of the ring finger. Of the remaining options, the median nerve is the main nerve of the forearm, supplying the majority of the flexor muscles of the anterior forearm (with two exceptions), thenar eminence and first two lumbricals; sensory innervation is to the volar thumb, index, middle and lateral half of the ring finger. The ulnar nerve innervates the remaining small muscles of the hand plus flexor carpi ulnaris and flexor digitorum profundus (medial); its sensory innervation is to the little finger and medial half of the ring finger. The axillary nerve supplies deltoid, triceps and teres minor; its sensory innervation is to the 'regimental patch' of the deltoid. The musculocutaneous nerve supplies upper arm muscles and sensory innervation to the lateral forearm. An effective way to rapidly assess the motor innervation of the nerves to the hand is by asking the patient to perform the hand motions of 'rock' (median nerve), 'paper' (radial nerve), 'scissors' (ulnar nerve) and 'OK' (anterior interosseous branch of the median nerve).

☑ 3d Apply U-slab or humeral brace, referral to orthopaedics

The application of a U-slab immobilises both the shoulder and elbow to aid splinting in the acute setting of the ED. A humeral brace functions in the same way and is preferred in younger patients with larger muscle bulk. The orthopaedic team should review the patient prior to discharge to determine follow-up and/or operative management. The majority of humeral shaft fractures are managed non-operatively, with up to 20 degrees angulation and 3–5 cm shortening being acceptable in many cases with little functional impairment. Successful union rates are as high as 90%. Operative management with open reduction and internal fixation (ORIF) may be required if adequate alignment cannot be maintained, or in the presence of open fractures, neurovascular injury, compartment syndrome, segmental fracture, polytrauma or a pathological fracture.

KEY LEARNING POINTS

- A good working knowledge of anatomy including neurovascular structures is essential when assessing any patient.
- When testing and documenting nerve function, it is essential to be specific to the individual nerve function and sensory pattern.
- Humeral fractures, in the absence of neurovascular injury, can successfully be treated non-operatively with humeral braces or a plaster slab with union rates as high as 90%.

My legs gave way

A 34-year-old man of South-East Asian descent presents to the emergency department after a collapse at home. He describes waking up with generalised myalgia and when he went to get out of bed, his legs gave way from underneath him. He lives alone and was unable to get himself up off the floor and so called an ambulance for help. He denies dizziness, light-headedness, chest pain or headache before the collapse and did not lose consciousness. He has had some minor muscle cramps and intermittent palpitations over the last few weeks but otherwise has been generally well. He has no past medical history or family history.

Lower limb neurological examination:

1. Power 2/5 at hip flexion, 4/5 distal lower limb
2. Increased tone and brisk reflexes bilaterally

Upper limb neurological examination:

1. Power 3/5 shoulder abduction, 5/5 distal upper limb bilaterally
2. Normal tone and reflexes bilaterally

An ECG is performed as part of the work-up.

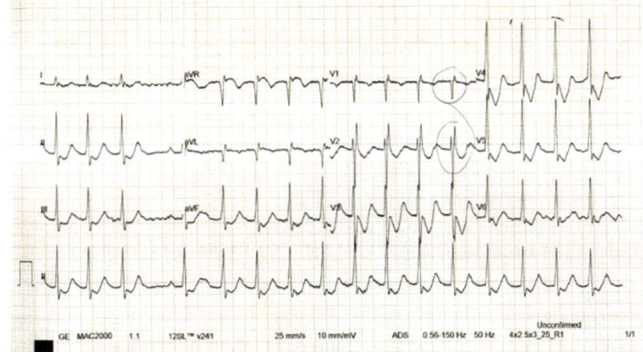

DOI: 10.1201/9781003461456-42

1.   Which of the following best describes the findings that are evident?

a.   Narrow complex tachycardia, widespread ST depression

b.   Prolonged PR interval, incomplete right bundle branch block (RBBB), U waves

c.   Incomplete RBBB and prolonged QTc

d.   Sinus tachycardia, prolonged QTc, U waves

e.   Prolonged PR interval, prolonged QTc, widespread ST depression

A venous blood gas (VBG) is performed which is shown.

⊙ POCT VENOUS BLOOD GAS

Component

Ref Range & Units				
Source	Venous	**Total Haemoglobin** g/l	161	
pH	7.395	**Deoxyhaemoglobin** %	23.6^	
Carbon Dioxide Partial Pressure kPa	6.17^	Comment: Value above reference range		
Comment: Value above reference range		**Oxyhaemoglobin** %	74.1ᵥ	
Oxygen Partial Pressure kPa	5.37ᵥ	Comment: Value below reference range		
Comment: Value below reference range		**Saturated Oxygen** %	75.8	
Potassium mmol/L	1.5ᵥ	**Carboxyhaemoglobin** %	1.4	
Comment: Value below reference range		**Methaemoglobin** %	0.9	
Sodium mmol/L	142	**Bilirubin** micromol/l	0ᵥ	
Ionised Calcium mmol/L	1.20	Comment: Value below reference range		
Chloride mmol/L	103	**Standard Base Excess** mmol/L	3.4^	
Glucose mmol/L	7.0^	Comment: Value above reference range		
Comment: Value above reference range		**Standard Bicarbonate** mmol/L	26.1	
Lactate mmol/L	2.5^	**Haematocrit** %	49.5	
Comment: Value above reference range		**Oxygen Tension at 50% Saturation** kPa	3.53	
Urea mmol/L	4.6	**Oxygen Content** mmol/L	7.5	
Creatinine micromol/l	52.0ᵥ			
Comment: Value below reference range				

A peripheral 18G cannula is in situ.

2. Which of the following is the most suitable initial replacement options for this patient?

    a. 40 mmol potassium chloride in 1 litre 0.9% sodium chloride IV over 4 hours

    b. 40 mmol potassium chloride in 1 litre 0.9% sodium chloride IV over 2 hours

    c. 40 mmol potassium chloride in 500 mL 0.9% sodium chloride IV over 1 hour

    d. 40 mmol potassium chloride in 100 mL 0.9% sodium chloride IV over 1 hour

    e. Sando-K® 12 mmol/tablet, 2 tablets, three times per day

You review the laboratory blood results.

RENAL PROFILE			ENDOCRINOLOGY		
Sodium	140		Free T3		
Potassium	1.7	v	Free T4	74.7	^
Urea			Thyroid stimulatin…	<0.01	v
Creatinine	59	v	**FULL BLOOD COUNT**		
Estimated GFR	>90*		Haemoglobin (g/L)	154	
LIVER PROFILE			MCV	82.6	
Alanine transaminase	36		HCT	0.462	
Albumin	42		White cell count	12.27	^
Alkaline phosphatase	173	^	Neutrophils	10.44	^
Bilirubin (total)	6		Lymphocytes	1.17	v
BONE PROFILE			Monocytes	0.60	
Calcium	2.32		Eosinophils	0.04	
Calcium (Albumin-a…	2.39		Basophils	0.02	
Phosphate	0.50	v	Platelet count	210	
CARDIAC PROFILE			MPV	9.2	
Cardiac Troponin T	7		MCH	27.5	
C-reactive protein	<0.6		MCHC (g/L)	333	
CHEMISTRY PROFILE			Red cell count	5.59	
Anti-TSH-receptor…			RDW	11.9	
Cortisol	793 *		XE Nucleated RBCs %	0.0	
Magnesium	0.74		XE Nucleated RBCs…	0.00	

3. Which of the following is the most likely diagnosis?

    a. Hypokalaemic periodic paralysis

    b. Renal tubular acidosis

    c. Guillain–Barré syndrome

    d. Primary hypoaldosteronism

    e. Thyrotoxic periodic paralysis

☑ **1b Prolonged PR interval, incomplete RBBB, U waves**

This ECG shows a number of abnormalities. Working through your ECG interpretation systematically will help to identify these. The rate is ~100 bpm, sinus rhythm, normal axis. The PR interval is prolonged (best seen in rhythm strip lead II) indicating 1st degree AV block, there is incomplete RBBB (RSR' V1-V3 with QRS duration <120 ms), prominent U waves (best seen in V2 and V3) with apparent QT elongation due to fusion of T waves with U waves leading to a long QU interval. These features together with the widespread ST depression and T-wave inversion are indicative of hypokalaemia and should make you be very concerned! With worsening hypokalaemia, you may begin to see frequent supraventricular and ventricular ectopic beats, supraventricular tachyarrhythmias (for example, atrial fibrillation [AF], atrial flutter, atrial tachycardia) and the potential to develop life-threatening ventricular arrhythmias such as ventricular tachycardia, ventricular fibrillation and torsades de pointes.

☑ **2b 40 mmol potassium chloride in 1 litre 0.9% sodium chloride IV over 2 hours**

For severe hypokalaemia (<2.5 mmol/L) or any ECG changes/cardiac instability or if symptomatic, treatment must be commenced immediately. The patient must be in a high-dependency area i.e. the resuscitation room on a cardiac monitor. In a mild to moderate hypokalaemia, peripheral intravenous replacement is generally maximum concentration of 40 mmol potassium per litre at a rate of 10 mmol/hour. However, it is generally recognised that in severe hypokalaemia, the rate that can be increased to 20 mmol/hour peripherally as long as cardiac monitoring is in place and the patient remains stable. Concentrated potassium (20–40 mmol/100 mL) can be used when there is risk of fluid overload and should only be given via a central line. 40 mmol/500 mL should ideally be given via a central line also, but can be given via a large-bore peripheral line pending central access if K <2.5 or <3.5 with cardiac instability which is likely to resolve with rapid replacement. The maximum rate of 20 mmol/hour still applies; only in a peri-arrest scenario with life-threatening arrhythmia, can concentrated potassium chloride be used at a higher rate. Ensure to check and replace magnesium as required as this provides more rapid correction of the hypokalaemia. Oral Sando-K® is not appropriate in severe hypokalaemia with ECG changes.

☑ **3e Thyrotoxic periodic paralysis**

Hypokalaemic periodic paralysis is a rare disorder characterised by potentially fatal episodes of muscle weakness and paralysis that can affect all muscles, including extra-ocular and respiratory musculature. It can be precipitated by exercise, stress or conditions associated with increased release of adrenaline, cortisol, aldosterone or insulin. Thyrotoxic periodic paralysis is a similar presentation in the context of thyrotoxicosis and the correct answer in this case as indicated by the thyroid function tests. Excess T4/T3 increases Na^+–K^+–ATPase activity and may increase susceptibility to the hypokalaemic action of adrenaline or insulin. Guillain–Barré is a rapidly progressive ascending paralysis that can be precipitated by illnesses such as gastroenteritis (which may itself cause K^+ loss); however, the clinical history and examination findings of proximal weakness do not fit this. Renal tubular acidosis encompasses three types that affect the kidney's ability to acidify urine, leading to a metabolic acidosis. Primary hypoaldosteronism is a cause of hyperkalaemia.

KEY LEARNING POINTS

- One of the most overlooked symptoms of hypokalaemia is muscle weakness and fatigue.
- ECG changes of severe hypokalaemia include prolongation of the PR interval, prolongation of the QT interval and the formation of U waves.
- In extreme circumstances, you can double the standard peripheral IV potassium chloride (KCl) infusion rate to 20 mmol per hour.
- Severe hyperthyroidism may rarely result in periodic hypokalaemia and paralysis.

CASE 43

Off legs

A 24-year-old man presents to the emergency department (ED) at 2300 hours following a fall at home where he was unable to get up, even with assistance of his parents. He describes a 3-month history of gradual motor and sensory neurological decline leading to this event. On further questioning, he states that he has been dropping items, having difficulties feeding himself and has been walking 'like a drunk'. Past medical history includes a pituitary adenoma recently diagnosed at another hospital in UK for which he takes daily oral steroid replacement. He reports that he has used cocaine and tobacco recreationally in the past but is currently using something called *Whippits* in an inhaled form.

Initial observations are recorded as HR 87, BP 128/74, SpO$_2$ 100% on room air, temperature 37.2°C (99.0°F), GCS 15/15. Neurological examination reveals significant ataxia, dysmetria, dysdiadochokinesia affecting upper and lower limbs, left more than right, with associated reduced power throughout (MRC 4/5).

ECG shows normal sinus rhythm.

1. Which further investigations and/or referrals are warranted in the ED overnight?
    a. Draw bloods (FBC/U&Es/CRP/coagulation profile), CT head with intracranial angiogram
    b. Draw bloods (FBC/U&Es/CRP/coagulation profile), MRI whole spine, referral to local neurosurgeons
    c. Draw bloods (FBC/U&Es/CRP), non-contrast CT head, referral to infectious diseases team
    d. Draw bloods (FBC/U&Es/CRP/coagulation profile), no imaging overnight, referral to acute internal medicine team
    e. Draw bloods (FBC/U&Es/CRP), no imaging overnight, referral to liaison mental health team

Further neurological findings on re-examination include saccadic eye movements and sensory disturbance to vibration in a glove & stocking distribution. The remaining cranial nerve examination is normal.

DOI: 10.1201/9781003461456-43

The patient is admitted and further imaging performed.

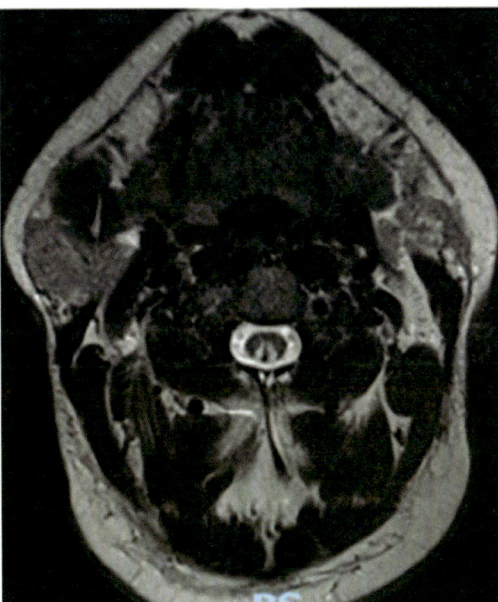

2. What is the best description of the appearances on this T2-weighted MRI?

   a. There is significant diffuse oedema within and beyond the dura

   b. Normal appearances of the spinal cord at this level

   c. There is asymmetric, hyperintense signal abnormality along the right spinothalamic tract and suggestion of subtle cervical cord swelling with contrast enhancement

   d. There is marked hyperintense signal abnormality along the cerebrospinal tracts and suggestion of subtle cervical cord swelling and contrast enhancement

   e. There is symmetrical bilateral hyperintense signal abnormality along the dorsal columns with the suggestion of subtle cervical cord swelling

The following laboratory blood test results are obtained for the patient.

FBC and Differential

Component	
Ref Range & Units	
White Cell Count	10.44^
3.0 - 10.0 x 10⁹/L	
Red Cell Count	4.88
4.4 - 5.8 x 10¹²/L	
Haemoglobin (g/L)	126ᵥ
130 - 170 g/L	
HCT	0.412
0.37 - 0.50 L/L	
MCV	84.4
80 - 99 fL	
MCH	25.8ᵥ
27.0 - 33.5 pg	
MCHC (g/L)	306ᵥ
320 - 360 g/L	
RDW	15.4^
11.5 - 15.0 %	
Platelet Count	404^
150 - 400 x 10⁹/L	
MPV	10.0
7 - 13 fL	
Neutrophils	6.21
2.0 - 7.5 x 10⁹/L	
Lymphocytes	3.05
1.2 - 3.65 x 10⁹/L	
Monocytes	1.10^
0.2 - 1.0 x 10⁹/L	
Eosinophils	0.06
0.0 - 0.4 x 10⁹/L	
Basophils	0.02
0.0 - 0.1 x 10⁹/L	
XE Nucleated RBCs Abs	0.00
0 - 0.01 x 10⁹/L	
XE Nucleated RBCs %	0.0

Plasma Methylmalonate

Component	
Ref Range & Units	
Plasma Methylmalonate	0.15
0 - 0.28 umol/L	

Comment: Plasma MMA values of less than 0.29 umol/L are considered not indicative of B12 deficiency.

(!) **Vitamin B12 & Serum Folate**

Component	
Ref Range & Units	
Vitamin B12	115ᵥ
197 - 771 pg/mL	
Serum Folate	7.0
2.9 - 26.8 ng/mL	

Comment: If no change in dietary habits, a normal serum folate makes folate deficiency unlikely.

3. Which of the following is the most likely underlying cause for the presentation in this patient?

   a. Pernicious anaemia

   b. Nitrous oxide abuse

   c. Vegan diet

   d. Proton pump inhibitor use

   e. Crohn's disease

☑ 1a Draw bloods (FBC/U&Es/CRP/coagulation profile), CT head with intracranial angiogram

This young man does have a known pituitary adenoma and, as there is no previous information available to guide acute management, a CT head to rule out obvious bleed or expanding lesion (for example, apoplexy) causing immediate pressure-related intracranial changes is sensible. However, in this case given the evident neurological deficit, early discussion with the stroke or neurology team and a CT head with CT angiogram would be beneficial to additionally exclude an ischaemic event or vertebral artery dissection, which are an important cause of 'strokes' in the under 45-year-old age group and may be related to athletic activity or exercise. If these are negative, he will need further investigation with MRI of the head and/or spine, but this would not be done out of hours overnight in most centres. The exception to this would be MRI lumbar spine for suspected cauda equina which is a time-critical diagnosis.

☑ 2e There is symmetrical bilateral hyperintense signal abnormality along the dorsal columns with the suggestion of subtle cervical cord swelling

On T2-weighted MRI, the signal intensifies where water and fat molecules accumulate, possibly indicating areas/lesions that are inflammatory (oedematous). Normal T2-weighted images of the spinal cord in cross-section views would demonstrate 'greyish' grey matter and darker white matter (as it is hypointense compared to grey matter). The image slice of the patient shows inflammatory changes along the dorsal columns of the spinal cord that light up as bright white, illustrating the 'inverted "V" sign'. This sign is commonly associated with subacute combined degeneration of the spinal cord, usually beginning at the thoracic level with ascending or descending progression. Lateral corticospinal tracts and sometimes lateral spinothalamic tract can also be involved. There are also often cerebral white matter changes. The dorsal column carries sensory modalities of fine touch, vibration and proprioception. First-order neurones carry sensory information from peripheral nerves to medulla oblongata travelling within the dorsal columns within the spinal cord. Second-order neurones decussate within the medulla oblongata and travel to the contralateral medial lemniscus to the thalamus. Lastly, the third-order neurons travel through the internal capsule to the ipsilateral primary sensory cortex.

☑ 3b Nitrous oxide abuse

The diagnosis is subacute combined degeneration of the cord. In this case, *Whippets* (street name for canisters of nitrous oxide or laughing gas) were being abused, leading to generation of nitrogen and oxygen free radicals that directly inactivate vitamin B12, which is a crucial cofactor for essential enzymes involved in maintaining healthy myelin.

All of the options are potential causes or precipitants of B12 deficiency, but most would also cause a concurrent anaemia. If there was no history of drug use and normal B12 levels, other differentials for the presentation include other nutritional or metabolic deficiencies (copper, vitamin E, methotrexate-induced myelopathy), demyelination secondary to multiple sclerosis or transverse myelitis, infection such as tabes dorsalis (tertiary syphilis) or cerebellar stroke. The treatment for subacute combined degeneration of the cord is vitamin B12 replacement, for example hydroxocobalamin 1 mg IM daily on alternate days until neurological improvement, then 1 mg IM every 2–3 months. Alternatively, oral administration can be sufficient once symptoms have resolved unless the deficiency is due to malabsorption, where parenteral administration must be continued.

KEY LEARNING POINTS

- Cranial imaging should be considered in cases where there are significant neurological findings. Be cautious of using age as a discriminating factor for certain pathology processes such as stroke.
- MRI is very sensitive for picking up radiological signs of subacute combined degeneration of the cord with a classical inverted V sign typically most prominent in the upper thoracic or lower cervical cord.
- Ask carefully about recreational drug use as part of routine history-taking as some patients may not ascribe their symptoms to chronic misuse and social acceptance.

Out of hospital cardiac arrest

A 55-year-old man is brought into the emergency department following an out of hospital cardiac arrest. The patient had been found unconscious by friends who performed bystander CPR. On the arrival of the ambulance crew, the initial rhythm was asystole. Interventions at the scene included 500 mL bolus of IV crystalloid, 4 rounds of 1 mg IV adrenaline and a total of 1.6 mg of IV naloxone. There was return of spontaneous circulation (ROSC) after 27 minutes.

On arrival to hospital, a primary survey is performed:

1. Airway: intubated and attached to an Oxylog ventilator
2. Breathing: SpO_2 98% with FiO_2 50%, irregular spontaneous respiratory effort, SIMV, TV 500 mL, Ppeak 28, PEEP 5, $ETCO_2$ 4.7 kPa, irregular spontaneous respiratory effort
3. Circulation: HR 110, BP 220/110, cool peripherally to elbows, 2 x IV cannulae in situ
4. Disability: GCS 3/15 (no sedation given by ambulance crew), pupils bilaterally dilated to 5 mm and poorly reactive to light
5. Exposure: soft abdomen, temperature 34°C (93.2°F), no external evidence of injury

Once stable, the patient is transferred for a non-contrast CT head scan.

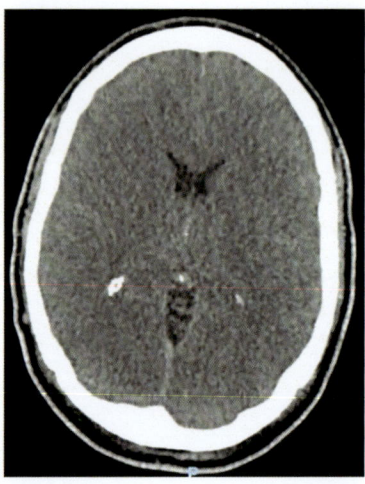

DOI: 10.1201/9781003461456-44

1. Which of the following is the best description of the CT findings?

    a. Subarachnoid haemorrhage (SAH)

    b. Global hypoxic brain injury

    c. Transverse sinus thrombosis

    d. Subdural haemorrhage

    e. No abnormality seen

Further history from the patient's friend is that the patient had been drinking alcohol and had taken approximately 600 mg of pregabalin. A point-of-care toxicology screen is positive for opioids, cocaine and benzodiazepines.

The intensive care unit (ICU) registrar suggests a dose of flumazenil to aid spontaneous ventilation.

2. Which of the following is the appropriate dose of flumazenil to give?

    a. 50 mcg IV, followed by 25 mcg every minute

    b. 100 mcg IV, followed by 50 mcg every minute

    c. 150 mcg IV, followed by 75 mcg every minute

    d. 200 mcg IV, followed by 75 mcg every minute

    e. No dose, flumazenil is not indicated

The patient has returned from CT and the following actions are completed:

1. The patient is settled onto a continuous propofol infusion
2. A urethral urinary catheter is inserted
3. Maintenance IV fluids are commenced
4. A 12-lead ECG is performed
5. A portable chest radiograph is performed

The ICU registrar suggests commencing the 'neuro-protective bundle' prior to transfer to the ICU.

3. Which of the following measures is the best description of a neuro-protective intervention?

    a. 70-degrees head-up position and loose endotracheal tube (ETT) tie

    b. Fraction of inspired oxygen 100%

    c. $PaCO_2$ target of 4.5 kPa

    d. IV methylprednisolone

    e. MAP >75 mmHg

☑ 1b Global hypoxic brain injury

The scan shows diffuse loss of grey-white differentiation of the cerebral and cerebellar hemispheres consistent with severe hypoxic ischaemic injury post-cardiac arrest. The key to this image is to appreciate it in clinical context; although the blood pressure is elevated suggesting a primary intracranial cause, the key abnormalities are the total loss of normal cerebral gyrus patterns, loss of grey-white matter differentiation and total effacement of the lateral ventricles. There is a suggestion of the classical 'starfish' pattern resembling SAH but in this case, it is due to global hypoxic injury and is called pseudosubarachnoid haemorrhage (PSAH). PSAH may also be seen in meningitis, dural venous sinus thrombosis, massive bilateral acute subdural haematoma (SDH) and with intra-thecal contrast. It has a density of 30–40 Hounsfield units (HU) whereas true SAH is closer to 60 HU.

☑ 2e No dose, flumazenil is not indicated

Flumazenil is only licensed for use for the reversal of sedative effects of benzodiazepines administrated in anaesthesia, intensive care and other clinical procedures where iatrogenic benzodiazepines have been given. Its use is contraindicated in patients with benzodiazepine dependency, signs of tricyclic antidepressant overdose, epilepsy controlled with benzodiazepines and mixed overdoses. In mixed overdoses if the benzodiazepine is reversed it may precipitate seizures which can be extremely difficult to control. Flumazenil is a competitive benzodiazepine antagonist. It competitively inhibits the activity of benzodiazepine and non-benzodiazepine substances that interact with benzodiazepine receptor site on the GABA/benzodiazepine receptor complex. When used it is given intravenously, the initial dose is 200 mcg over 15 seconds followed by 100 mcg every 1 minute if required with a maximum dose of 1 mg.

☑ 3c $PaCO_2$ target of 4.5 kPa

The neuro-protective bundle refers to a set of measures that are designed to reduce the risk of developing secondary brain injury. These include: head 30-degrees up with the ETT taped or loosely tied (helps with cerebral venous drainage); low normocapnia with a $PaCO_2$ of 4.5 to 5 kPa and avoidance of hypoxia with a PaO_2 of >8 kPa (regulates cerebral blood flow within autoregulatory range); target systolic blood pressure above 90 mmHg or MAP >65 mmHg (helps with maintaining cerebral perfusion pressure); analgesia and sedation (reduces total brain metabolic demand). Other more invasive and specific measures also include intracranial pressure (ICP) monitoring and cerebral oxygenation monitoring. Methylprednisolone, although it might help with cerebral oedema transiently, has not been shown to improve long-term outcomes and may be deleterious due to its effects on blood sugar.

KEY LEARNING POINTS

- Post-global hypoxic injury CT appearances may mimic early signs of subarachnoid haemorrhage. Seek advice from a neuroradiologist to clarify indeterminate cases.
- Flumazenil is only licensed for pure benzodiazepine overdose and may precipitate seizures in mixed overdoses.
- Be aware of the components of the neuro-protective bundle as it can be easily instituted in the ED whilst awaiting transfer to ICU or a neurosurgical unit.

CASE 45

Packing, stuffing, pushing

A 56-year-old man is brought to the emergency department (ED) from an international railway station accompanied by Border Force agents having arrived from Amsterdam. He was initially stopped due to not completing the health questionnaire but was then found to have traces of cocaine on his clothes and traces of cocaine, heroin and spice on his belongings. He is suspected of ingestion of drug packages but a scanner at the station was 'inconclusive'. He denies any symptoms.

Initial observations are all within normal limits, he appears tearful and slightly anxious but not overtly agitated.

1. As the triage clinician, which of the following is the best initial management?
   a. Gain verbal consent, draw bloods (FBC/U&Es), ECG, stream to majors for intimate examination and removal of packages
   b. Gain verbal consent, draw bloods (FBC/U&Es), ECG, redirect to urgent treatment centre for observation
   c. Gain verbal consent, draw bloods for VBG, ECG, consider low-dose CT abdomen & pelvis, stream to majors for clinical review
   d. Gain verbal consent, draw bloods (FBC/U&Es), ECG, abdominal radiograph, stream to majors for clinical review
   e. Gain verbal consent, draw bloods (FBC/U&Es), ECG, urinary drug screen, stream to majors for 8 hours of observation

The Border Force officers present a document to you with a signed request from a high-ranking officer that states that you must perform an immediate radiograph or ultrasound to look for ingested drugs under the Police and Criminal Act 1984 (PACE), section 55A, subsection 1.

You show the patient the document and the patient refuses to consent to this as he is worried about the radiation dose.

2. What would you do next?
   a. Proceed to plain abdominal radiograph without patient consent
   b. Arrange an urgent ultrasound to mitigate the radiation risk
   c. Convince the patient to consent to the procedure as it will speed up discharge
   d. Advise the officers that you cannot proceed against patient consent
   e. Proceed to CT abdomen & pelvis with contrast as the definitive imaging modality without patient consent

DOI: 10.1201/9781003461456-45

The man remains asymptomatic in the department and is noted by officers to have passed a packet.

He then consents to investigation.

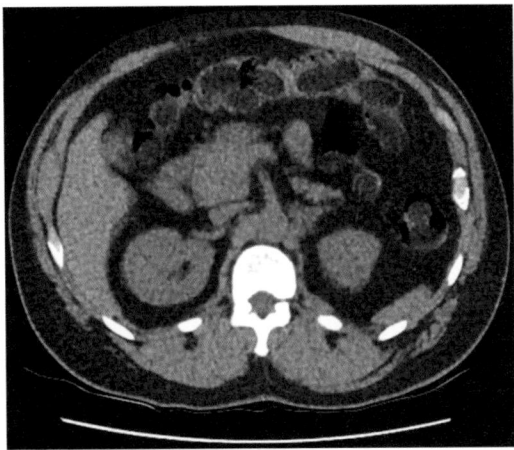 

3. Based on the imaging, what would your next step be?

    a. Discharge after 4 hours' observation in the ED

    b. Admit for 8 hours' observation under the acute internal medicine team

    c. Discharge to the custody of the Border Forces with a sealed discharge summary for the receiving medical officer

    d. Discharge after 2 hours' observation in the ED

    e. Discharge to the custody of the Border Forces without any documentation

☑ 1c Gain verbal consent, draw bloods for VBG, ECG, consider low-dose CT abdomen & pelvis, stream to majors for clinical review

Suspected internal drug traffickers are divided into three types: body packers (professionally packed, high number of packages, usually detained by Border Forces, lower risk of rupture but catastrophic if they do); body stuffers (usually cling-film wraps, swallowed quickly to conceal on arrest, higher risk of rupture and absorption); and body pushers (well packaged items inserted into cavities to smuggle drugs, low risk of rupture). This patient is likely to be a body packer or 'drug mule' based on location of arrest at an international railway station. A full set of observations and ECG are recommended along with blood glucose as a minimum investigation set. Further laboratory bloods are not generally indicated unless drug toxidrome symptoms are present according to current UK guidelines. Urinary drug screens are difficult to interpret as the patient may also have 'used' drugs and this may falsely guide you. Also, it may not necessarily indicate the type of drug ingested as it may not have leaked out. Do not try and retrieve drug packets in the ED due to risk of rupture and potentially severe consequences from absorption.

☑ 2d Advise the officers that you cannot proceed against patient consent

Current advice from the Royal College of Emergency Medicine UK (May 2020), states that clinicians are not required to perform abdominal radiograph or ultrasound scan even when presented with a written request under PACE, section 55A. In addition, plain radiographs or ultrasound are no longer recommended for the investigation of suspected drug packet ingestion. Low-dose CT (as used in CT KUB) is the recommended modality of choice. This should be reported by a senior radiologist and is helpful in cases where multiple packages are suspected to have been ingested. They can be considered in body stuffers but be aware that there is a higher false-negative rate as the number of packages is typically few and they are poorly packaged making them hard to identify. The total radiation dose from low-dose CT is about 3 mSv, which is equivalent to 1 year's background radiation in the UK and the lifetime additional risk of fatal cancer per examination around 1 in 10 000.

☑ 3c Discharge to the custody of the Border Forces with a sealed discharge summary for the receiving medical officer

The low-dose CT shown above confirms the presence of multiple drug packages distributed throughout the entire bowel and into the rectum. Typically, body packers can carry up to 1 kg of drugs, with cocaine and heroin being the most frequently packed drugs. As this patient is asymptomatic and has passed a package, he may be discharged into the custody of the Border Forces. Do not handle any passed packages and allow the Border Forces to maintain the chain of evidence. The Border Forces will place the patient into highly observed custody and wait until the patient has passed the rest of the packages. Good practice mandates that the patient is discharged with a written discharge summary in a sealed envelope. Body stuffers (street dealers, wraps) are at high risk of rupture and should, in general, be observed for 8 hours from suspected ingestion under the acute internal medicine team. In case of systemic toxicity, consult appropriate local toxicology guidelines, for example in the UK, Toxbase from the National Poisons Information Service, move to the resuscitation room and initiate treatment according to suspected drug. These patients may need emergency surgery to retrieve packages.

KEY LEARNING POINTS

- Routine blood testing and urinary toxicology screening for drugs of abuse is not recommended for the majority of asymptomatic patients who are suspected of ingesting drug packages.
- Patients must consent to investigation and cannot be forced to do so against their will if they display capacity to make those decisions.
- Stable patients with well-packaged drugs ('drug mules') may be discharged into the custody of Border Force agents who have specialist units where patients may pass the rest of the packages.

Palpitations

A 45-year-old woman self-presents to the emergency department (ED) complaining of palpitations for the last 90 minutes. She denies any other associated symptoms, such as chest pain, dizziness or shortness of breath. She denies any past medical history. A member of nursing staff approaches you as they note the pulse oximeter reads the heart rate as 200 bpm, but on palpating the pulse they did not believe this was a true reading.

You call the patient through to assess them as part of the Rapid Assessment and Treatment team. On examination, initial observations are HR approximately 200 (manually recorded with regular radial pulse), BP 127/94, SpO$_2$ 99% on room air, RR 16, temperature 37.1°C (98.8°F), GCS 15/15. She looks well, is warm peripherally with CRT <2 seconds and cardiorespiratory examinations are otherwise normal.

You move the patient to the resuscitation room, apply 3-lead ECG monitoring and defibrillator pads.

A 12-lead ECG is then performed.

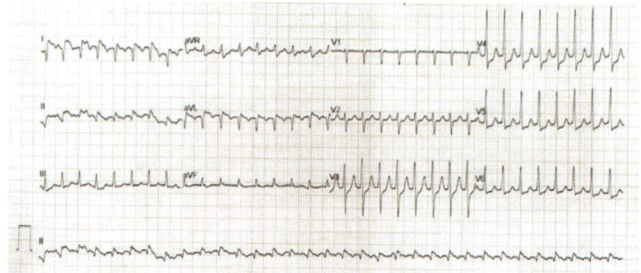 

1. Which of the following is the best management option at this stage?

   a. Give adenosine 6 mg IV

   b. Prepare for synchronised DC cardioversion at 100 J biphasic

   c. Give metoprolol 5 mg IV at 1 mg per minute

   d. Attempt vagal manoeuvres and if that fails give adenosine 6 mg IV

   e. Give a crystalloid fluid bolus (20 mL/kg) and magnesium sulfate 4 g over 30 minutes

DOI: 10.1201/9781003461456-46

A repeat ECG is performed following your intervention.

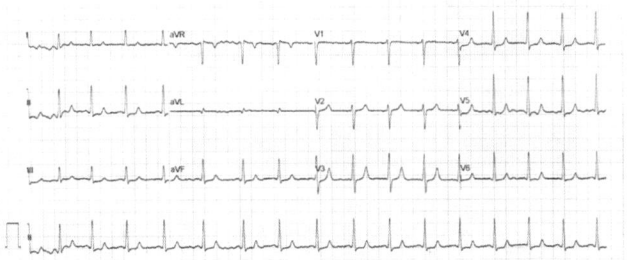 

2. What does this show?

    a. Normal sinus rhythm with early repolarisation

    b. Sinus rhythm with delta waves suggestive of Wolff–Parkinson–White

    c. Sinus rhythm with short PR interval

    d. Atrial flutter with a 3:1 block

    e. U waves

The patient remains well after a period of observation in the department and there is no evidence of reversion to the tachycardia.

3. Which of the following is the best option for further management?

    a. Discharge with cardiology electrophysiology outpatient follow-up and safety net advice

    b. Commence on oral dronedarone and discharge with cardiology outpatient follow-up and safety net advice

    c. Admit under the acute internal medicine team for cardiac monitoring, serial Troponins and inpatient cardiology consult

    d. Commence on digoxin 125 mcg OD and discharge with cardiology outpatient follow-up and safety net advice

    e. Commence on sotalol 40 mg BD and discharge with cardiology outpatient follow-up and safety net advice

☑ 1d Attempt vagal manoeuvres and if that fails give adenosine 6 mg IV

This ECG shows a regular, narrow QRS complex tachycardia with no P waves visualised, suggestive of a supraventricular tachycardia (SVT). Classifications of SVT are based on the pathway by which the electrical activity is taken from the atria: AV nodal re-entrant tachycardia (AVNRT) or AV re-entrant tachycardia (AVRT). This type of tachyarrhythmia is classified as a 'peri-arrest rhythm' based on the guidelines from the Resuscitation Council UK and therefore the patient should be moved to the appropriate area with suitable monitoring (including continuous 3-lead cardiac monitoring, pulse oximetry and bloods pressure monitoring) with defibrillator pads in situ. Before attempting cardioversion, you should also ensure to have sufficient staff available. Vagal manoeuvres should be attempted next and can include asking the patient to perform a Valsalva manoeuvre either by bearing down as if having a bowel movement or telling the patient to blow through the barrel of a 10 or 20 mL syringe for 15–20 seconds. Alternative vagal manoeuvres include cold stimulus to the face, forceful and sustained cough or triggering the gag reflex. Carotid massage can stimulate the vagal nerve but is associated with risk of stroke. Avoid this in older patients or those with atherosclerotic disease. The REVERT trial showed that a modified Valsalva with leg elevation after the strain phase increases likelihood of success from approximately 20% to 40%. If this fails, adenosine 6 mg IV should be administered. This should be into a large, well working cannula followed by a good saline flush as the half-life of adenosine is short (<10 seconds). If the 6 mg bolus fails, this can be repeated twice more at 12 mg and 18 mg. Synchronised DC cardioversion is indicated if there are adverse features, such as haemodynamic instability, chest pain, heart failure or syncope.

☑ 2c Sinus rhythm with short PR interval

The PR interval seen on this ECG is shortened, which is best seen in the lead II rhythm strip. Normal PR is 0.12–0.2 seconds i.e. 3–5 small squares but can be seen as 2–2.5 small squares in this trace. A short PR interval is suggestive of a pre-excitation syndrome. However, there is no slurred upstroke of the QRS complex which would indicate delta waves, nor a widened QRS complex (>0.12 seconds) that are indicative of Wolff–Parkinson–White syndrome. The presence of a shortened PR interval without these key features is sometimes referred to as Lown–Ganong–Levine syndrome (although this term is contentious). A short PR interval is also associated with junctional arrhythmias like AVNRT/AVRT or a near junctional rhythm, which is most likely in this case. The baseline is slightly 'wandering' but there is no sawtooth pattern suggestive of atrial flutter. Early repolarisation, also known as 'high take-off' or 'J-point elevation' is widespread concave ST elevation most prominent in the precordial leads seen in young healthy patients <50 years old. A U wave is a small deflection immediately after the T wave; prominent U waves are most commonly seen in bradycardia or severe hypokalaemia.

☑ 3a Discharge with cardiology electrophysiology outpatient follow-up and safety net advice

The best option here is to discharge but refer directly to the cardiology clinic for electrophysiology review for consideration of ablation. If symptoms are mild and infrequent, patients may be followed up without need for ablation or pharmacotherapy. Catheter ablation has been shown to have significant success rate in preventing tachyarrhythmia episodes compared to anti-arrhythmic drugs. However, if there are recurrent episodes whilst awaiting intervention, an anti-arrhythmic drug may be considered. Common medications include a calcium-channel blocker such as diltiazem or verapamil, or alternatively a beta-blocker such as bisoprolol. Note that diltiazem plus beta-blocker should be avoided, particularly in the elderly, due to increased risk of AV block. It is important to provide safety net advice regarding vagal manoeuvres and to return to the ED if symptoms return.

KEY LEARNING POINTS

- Follow standard ALS (or ACLS) management protocols for the management of tachyarrhythmias.
- A Valsalva manoeuvre followed by lifting the legs rapidly whilst supine on a bed may increase SVT cardioversion rate from 20% to 40% success.
- Patients can be considered for discharge post-cardioversion if they are cardiovascularly stable, have normal electrolytes and thyroid function and have no further episodes during observation in the ED.

Pleuritic chest pain

A 28-year-old woman presents to the emergency department (ED) complaining of sudden onset chest pain that she notes is most severe on deep inspiration. The pain started around 12 hours ago and has progressively worsened. She denies any other symptoms, including shortness of breath, cough or fever and she feels otherwise well in herself. She is a social smoker of cigarettes 2–3 times per week and there is no history of travel. There is no past medical history.

Initial observations are recorded as HR 60, BP 125/80, SpO$_2$ 98% on room air, RR 18, temperature 37.2°C (100°F).

A chest radiograph has been performed.

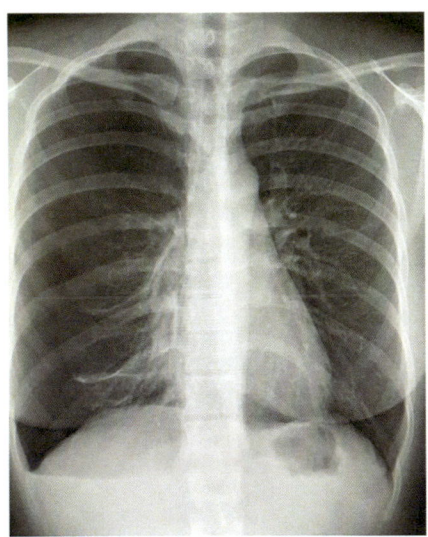

DOI: 10.1201/9781003461456-47

1. Based on the findings, which of the following is the best initial management of this patient?

   a. Administer broad-spectrum IV antibiotics, and perform a pleural aspirate and apply Light's criteria

   b. Administer high-flow O_2 via non-rebreathe mask and perform a needle aspiration in the 4th intercostal space, anterior to the mid-axillary line

   c. Administer high-flow O_2 via non-rebreathe mask and insert a small-bore chest drain (<14Fr) in the 4th intercostal space, mid-axillary line

   d. Administer high-flow O_2 via non-rebreathe mask and perform a needle decompression in 2nd intercostal space, mid-clavicular line

   e. Allow to use Entonox whilst preparing for needle aspiration in the 4th intercostal space, mid-axillary line

The patient's chest pain has improved following your intervention. Her observations all remain in normal range for the next 2 hours.

A repeat chest radiograph is performed.

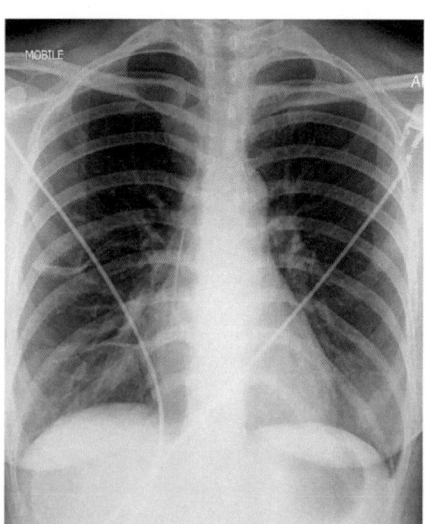

2. What is the best next management option?

   a. Continue high-flow oxygen, insert a small-bore chest drain (<14Fr) and refer to the acute internal medicine team

   b. Give oral co-codamol, allow the patient to use Entonox and review after 1 hour, discharge if the pain has resolved

   c. Consider discharge and refer for outpatient respiratory (pleural) appointment within 2–4 weeks, ensuring to advise patient to return if symptoms recur

   d. Continue high-flow oxygen and refer to the acute internal medicine team as this patient needs to be admitted for 24-hour observation

   e. Request a CT pulmonary angiogram to exclude underlying pulmonary embolus or interstitial lung injury

The patient's family lives in China and she was planning on arranging a visit in the next few weeks.

3. Which of the following is the advice you would give about flying and what other information would you provide?

   a. The patient can only fly 1 month after full clinical resolution, scuba diving is only permitted 6 months after full resolution, smoking cessation advice

   b. The patient can fly 1 week after full radiological resolution, scuba diving is contraindicated for life unless specialist assessment prior, smoking cessation advice

   c. The patient can fly 8 weeks after full clinical resolution, scuba diving is essentially contraindicated, recommend swapping to vaping

   d. The patient can only fly 6 weeks after full clinical resolution, scuba diving is essentially contraindicated, smoking cessation advice

   e. The patient should be recommended to travel at sea level for the next year, smoking cessation advice

☑ 1b Administer high-flow O$_2$ via non-rebreathe mask and perform a needle aspiration in the 4th intercostal space, anterior to the mid-axillary line

This chest radiograph shows a large right-sided pneumothorax with no mediastinal shift. As per the British Thoracic Society (BTS) guidelines, the pneumothorax should be measured from the hilum horizontally to the lung border. Using this method, this estimates the observed pneumothorax at approximately 3–4 cm. Given the history, this would be considered a large (>2 cm) primary spontaneous pneumothorax (PSP). Current guidelines from the BTS advise the initial management in these cases as needle aspiration. High-flow oxygen via a non-rebreathe mask provides a high FiO$_2$ that reduces the partial pressure of nitrogen in the pneumothorax and is thought to accelerate the resolution; caution should be taken in O$_2$ sensitive COPD patients. Entonox is contraindicated as this will convert the simple pneumothorax to a tension pneumothorax. If the patient is >50 years old with significant smoking history or has underlying lung disease, this is a secondary spontaneous pneumothorax (SSP), which are generally less well tolerated. In these cases, if the pneumothorax is 1–2 cm, needle aspiration is recommended; however, if the pneumothorax is >2 cm or the patient is breathless, insertion of a chest drain is recommended. When inserting a chest drain, take care to be just anterior to the mid-axillary line to avoid any damage to the long thoracic nerve of Bell.

☑ 2c Consider discharge and refer for outpatient respiratory (pleural) appointment within 2–4 weeks, ensuring to advise patient to return if symptoms recur

Needle aspiration was performed with 1.6 L of air aspirated before the repeat chest radiograph was performed. The repeat radiograph shows improved appearances with a small (~1 cm) apical pneumothorax remaining. Given that the pneumothorax is now less than 2 cm and her symptoms have improved, it is suitable to discharge from the ED and arrange follow-up with a respiratory outpatient appointment within 4 weeks. It is important to advise the patient to return if symptoms worsen to exclude re-accumulation of the pneumothorax. This patient was discharged and reviewed in the acute internal medicine ambulatory hot clinic around 1 week later for a repeat chest radiograph and referral to the pleural service. Insertion of a small-bore chest drain is recommended if needle aspiration fails (pneumothorax >2 cm and/or breathless); aspiration should not be repeated unless the procedure was performed incorrectly. Admission is not indicated in this setting as she felt well, her observations were normal and the pneumothorax had responded to needle aspiration. For a secondary pneumothorax the patient should generally be admitted for observation, particularly after needle aspiration given slower resolution and increased complication rate.

☑ 3b The patient can fly 1 week after full radiological resolution, scuba diving is contraindicated for life unless specialist assessment prior, smoking cessation advice

As per International Air Transport Association (IATA) & BTS Air Travel Working Group guidelines, patients with a PSP that has fully resolved can fly 1 week after full resolution. This is extended to 2 weeks for a traumatic pneumothorax. Do note that there are caveats to this if urgent air transfer is needed. The patient can travel before 7 days with a chest drain in situ as long as this has a Heimlich (one-way) valve in place. Reduced atmospheric partial pressure that occurs with increasing altitude during air travel leads to gas expansion; this means any residual pneumothorax could expand and cause a tension pneumothorax. Though airplane cabins are pressurised, this is still below atmospheric pressure at sea level. The same physiological process would occur if the patient were to ascend to high altitude on land. Full resolution would mean that the patient has had follow-up chest radiograph or CT chest that demonstrates that the lung has fully re-expanded. Scuba diving is contraindicated unless bilateral pleurectomies are performed with subsequent normal imaging and lung function tests post-operatively. Smokers are at higher risk of developing pneumothorax, but despite this the majority of young patients continue to smoke after their first episode of PSP. The risk of recurrence is as high as 50%. Vaping has also been shown to increase the risk of pneumothorax and should also be discouraged.

KEY LEARNING POINTS

- The BTS guidelines recommend pleural needle aspiration as a first line treatment in a stable patient with a large (>2 cm measured at the hilum) pneumothorax.
- High-flow oxygen therapy works by nitrogen washout and encourages lung re-expansion.
- Seek specialist advice regarding air travel and other activities post-pneumothorax and provide this information in both a verbal and written manner.
- Smoking and vaping cessation should be encouraged as both will increase the risk of pneumothorax recurrence.

POCUS

A 60-year-old woman presents to the emergency department after a passer-by sees her slumping on the seat at a bus stop. She declines to identify herself, provide history or allow physical examination. Her observations and capillary blood glucose performed with the ambulance service were normal. From the end of the bed, you observe multiple dry skin lesions and copious body lice across her person, and she appears confused.

After several hours, she agrees to basic blood tests. You are soon after alerted by the pathology laboratory of the following abnormal results: WCC 23, CRP 268 and blood cultures rapidly growing an organism suspicious for infective endocarditis.

A point-of-care ultrasound transthoracic echocardiogram (TTE) is performed.

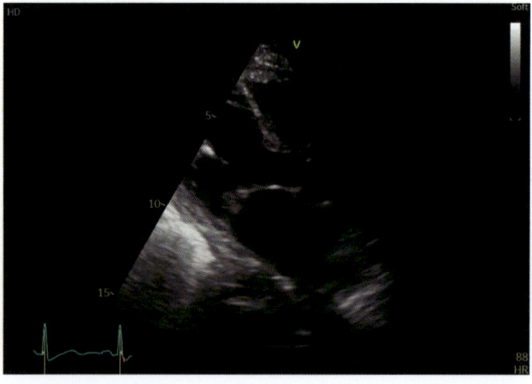 

1. Which standard TTE view is shown?

    a. Parasternal long axis (PLAX)

    b. Parasternal short axis (PSAX)

    c. Suprasternal

    d. Apical 5-chamber

    e. Subcostal 4-chamber

A further TTE view is obtained.

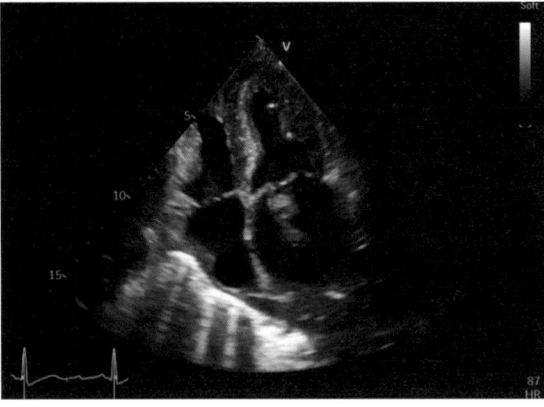

2. What is the main abnormality detected?

   a. Septal tricuspid valve leaflet vegetation

   b. Medial tricuspid valve leaflet vegetation

   c. Aortic valve leaflet vegetation

   d. Pulmonary valve leaflet vegetation

   e. Mitral valve leaflet vegetation

3. Which of the following organisms only requires to be isolated in a single blood culture sample to be sufficient to make the diagnosis of infective endocarditis?

   a. *Streptococcus mitis*

   b. *Staphylococcus epidermidis*

   c. *Coxiella burnetii*

   d. *Kingella kingae*

   e. *Eikenella corrodens*

☑ 1a Parasternal long axis (PLAX)

Echocardiography can be a complex and specialist area, but knowledge of some of the basic windows to enable ultrasound views is a good idea. European convention is image projection to start at the top of the screen with the shallowest structures uppermost, fanning out to display those lying deeper. The PLAX view, shown above, is excellent for looking at the anterior structures of the heart and is obtained with the patient in the left decubitus position using the phased array cardiac probe in the 3rd/4th intercostal space close to the left sternal edge. It is very good for showing the left ventricle and atrium, the mitral valve, the aortic valve and the outflow tract. The right ventricle is at the top of the image and incompletely visualised. The PSAX view is three levels: mid-papillary, mitral valve ('fish mouth') and aortic valve ('Mercedes-Benz sign') levels. The PSAX views provide further assessment of the left ventricle, mitral and aortic valves and right ventricular function. The apical 5-chamber view allows assessment of diastolic dysfunction, valvular regurgitation and cardiac output. The subcostal 4-chamber view is most often used as part of the eFAST scan protocol to rapidly assess for pericardial fluid but can also be used if apical views are technically difficult to achieve. The suprasternal view can be used in some situations, such as measuring aortic arch width, assessing for dissection or coarctation, or quantifying aortic regurgitation.

☑ 2e Mitral valve leaflet vegetation

On this apical 4-chamber view, you can appreciate a mobile irregular mass seen attached to the atrial side of the anterior mitral valve leaflet. In normal anatomy, the mitral valve has two leaflets: anterior and posterior. If we initially consider the first view (PLAX), you can see the mass clearly 'plopping' in and out with the cardiac cycle timed on the bottom left. This mass is then further augmented by the apical 4-chamber view, which confirms the relationship of the mass to the atrial side of the mitral valve on the right of the image. The right side of the heart appears normal and so the tricuspid valve, which has three leaflets (septal, anterior and posterior), is eliminated. The aortic and pulmonary valves cannot be visualised on the apical 4-chamber view, which excludes these options. On further imaging in this case, the parasternal 'fishmouth' short axis view would be useful to conclusively determine which leaflet (anterior or posterior) the vegetation is attached to. Vegetations are almost universally classified as small (<0.5 cm square), medium (0.5–1 cm square) or large (>1 cm square); this lesion is 4 cm square with a very high embolic risk.

☑ 3c *Coxiella burnetii*

Duke University Medical Center revised their 1994 diagnostic criteria for infective endocarditis in 2000 to produce the so-called 'modified Duke's criteria'. These changes are reflected in the European Society of Cardiology guidelines, with the addition of nuclear medicine and imaging criteria in 2015. To make a definite diagnosis of infective endo-carditis, one of the following must occur: two major criteria, OR one major + three minor criteria, OR five minor criteria satisfied (OR pathological diagnosis with culture or microscopy of a vegetation, embolism or intra-cardiac abscess). Major criteria include positive blood cultures for typical organisms from two separate samples and evidence of endocardial involvement such as echocardiogram evidence or new valvular regur-gitation. Minor criteria include predisposing heart condition or intravenous drug use, fever, embolic phenomena (arterial emboli, mycotic aneurysm, conjunctival haemor-rhage, Janeway's lesions), immunologic phenomena (glomerulonephritis, Osler's nodes, Roth's spots) or positive blood culture not meeting major criterion. Only *Coxiella bur-netii*, a Gram-negative, obligate intracellular bacterium responsible for Q ('Query') fever, requires a single positive culture (or serology) to count as a major criterion. Q fever was discovered following an outbreak amongst workers in an abattoir in Brisbane, Australia – it is extremely rare in the UK unless in exams!

KEY LEARNING POINTS

- Point-of-care echocardiography with focused windows is a useful adjunct for the acute or emergency physician and proficiency is recommended in four views – parasternal long axis, parasternal short axis, apical 4-chamber, subcostal 4-chamber.
- Valvular vegetations may be visualised if large enough and with a skilled operator. Remember that transoesophageal echocardiography has greater sensitivity than transthoracic.
- The modified Duke's criteria remain the gold standard for diagnosing infective endocarditis.

Right iliac fossa pain

A 17-year-old woman presents to the emergency department with her mother, complaining of a 5-day history of severe right iliac fossa pain with mild nausea. She states she has suffered with bloating over the past few months but denies any altered bowel habit. Her last menstrual period was 2 weeks ago and she denies any change in vaginal discharge or intermenstrual bleeding. She reports she is not sexually active. She had an appointment with her GP the day before, who noted a temperature of 38°C (100.4°F) with otherwise normal observations.

On examination, all observations are within normal limits, and she is afebrile. The abdomen is mildly distended, but soft with tenderness in the right iliac fossa without guarding.

1. Which of the following is the LEAST likely to be included in your initial differentials?
   a. Acute appendicitis
   b. Ectopic pregnancy
   c. Ovarian torsion
   d. Mesenteric adenitis
   e. Irritable bowel syndrome

A bedside point-of-care ultrasound performed by the emergency medicine registrar appears to show a fluid-filled mass.

DOI: 10.1201/9781003461456-49

A CT abdomen & pelvis is ordered, and the patient referred to a specialist team for further management.

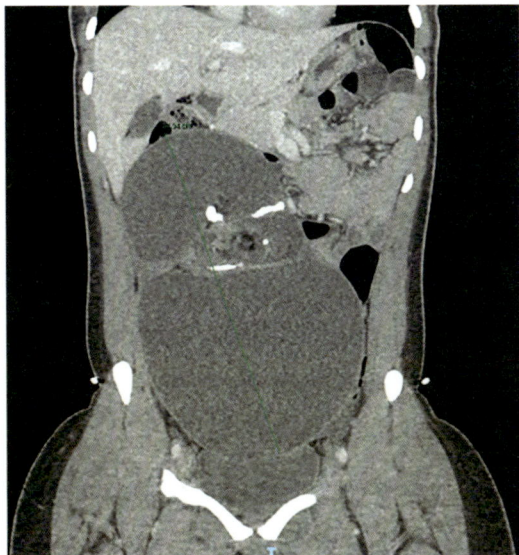

2. Based on the image provided, which of the following is the most likely diagnosis?
   a. Caecal volvulus causing large bowel obstruction
   b. Chronic appendicitis causing large bowel obstruction
   c. Ovarian dermoid cyst
   d. Hydatid cyst
   e. Ovarian torsion

3. What is the risk of malignant transformation associated with this diagnosis?
   a. 0.5–1%
   b. 1–2%
   c. 3–4%
   d. 5%
   e. 10%

☑ 1e Irritable bowel syndrome

The potential differential diagnosis for a young patient with right iliac fossa pain is wide, and all of the above could be considered in this case. However, the diagnosis of irritable bowel syndrome is generally a diagnosis of exclusion, particularly when there are other symptoms and signs that suggest a potential more serious cause. Acute abdominal pain with fever can be indicative of appendicitis. Mesenteric adenitis is characterised by right lower quadrant pain due to inflammation of the mesenteric lymph nodes, which commonly occurs after an upper respiratory tract infection; it is more common in the paediatric population. In any girl or woman of reproductive age, it is essential to exclude an ectopic pregnancy as a cause of her symptoms. Always perform a urinary β-hCG, even if sexual activity is denied (remember this is a teenager answering questions in front of her mother!). Ovarian torsion typically presents with very sudden and severe lower abdominal pain associated with nausea and vomiting. This can be preceded by intermittent pain for days to weeks beforehand due to twisting and untwisting. Though this case is not the typical history, it is certainly on the differential list.

☑ 2c Ovarian dermoid cyst

The CT slice shows a large generally homogenous mass arising from the pelvis, likely from the right side. There is some heterogeneity in the upper central portion with possible calcified elements present. This is most likely to be a large ovarian dermoid cyst with no evidence of torsion or rupture. Features on CT that suggest torsion include enlarged ovary, ovary shifted to midline, displaced uterus to involved side and fat stranding in the adnexa. Note that the definitive diagnosis of dermoid cyst requires histology. Although her pain was located to the right iliac fossa and she reported a brief history, the diagnosis in this case is clearly not acute appendicitis. CT findings in acute appendicitis are of increased appendiceal diameter with wall thickening and enhancement, intraluminal fluid and peri-appendiceal inflammation demonstrated by fat stranding, phlegmon or abscess. Hydatid cysts are caused by infection by the larval stage of the dog tapeworm. The liver is the most commonly affected organ; this mass is seen separately from the liver in this instance.

☑ 3b 1–2%

The most common complications of dermoid cysts include torsion and rupture. There is a small risk of malignant transformation, typically into squamous cell carcinoma (adults), though in the paediatric population this can also be endodermal sinus tumours. It is difficult to diagnose malignant transformation pre-operatively unless there is invasion into adjacent structures. It is more common in post-menopausal women and has a worse prognosis than primary malignant neoplasms of the ovary. Other complications of dermoid cysts include infection, carcinoid syndrome and paraneoplastic anti-NMDA receptor associated limbic encephalitis.

KEY LEARNING POINTS

- Point-of-care ultrasound can be a useful adjunct in assessing patients with abdominal pain. Care must be taken to use it in a rule-in strategy and there must be adequate governance procedures for image review.
- Ovarian dermoid cysts are a type of germ-cell tumour and often are not symptomatic until they reach a certain size and cause mass effect or complications such as torsion.
- There is a 1–2% risk of malignant transformation.

CASE 50

Right upper quadrant pain

A 39-year-old man presents to the emergency department (ED) overnight complaining of worsening pain in his upper abdomen over the last 48 hours. He describes the pain as intermittent and colicky, radiating around the right flank to the back and is associated with nausea. He denies a change in bowel habit, has not had diarrhoea or vomiting, nor fever. At time of assessment, he has already received 10 mg morphine intravenously and he reports the pain is still 6/10. He had a previous partial hepatectomy due to hydatid disease with biliary reconstruction a few years ago and immune thrombocytopenia (ITP) for which he takes no treatment.

Initial observations are all within normal limits. He is warm and well perfused with CRT <2 seconds. Cardiorespiratory examinations are normal. On palpation of the abdomen, he is tender in the right upper quadrant with local guarding, but the remainder of the abdomen is soft.

The following imaging is performed.

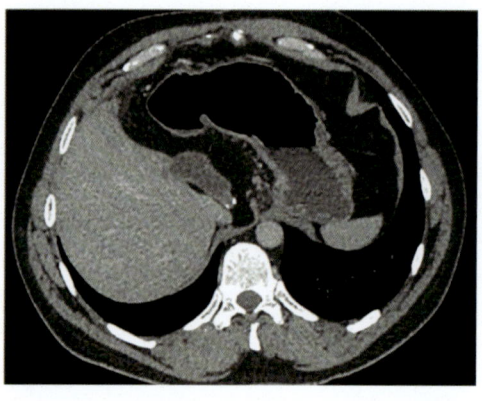 

1. Which of the following seen on the image could best account for patient's symptoms?
   a. Biliary duct dilatation
   b. Large bowel obstruction
   c. Biliary stone
   d. Recurrence of hydatid disease
   e. Gastric cancer

DOI: 10.1201/9781003461456-50

2. Which of the following imaging modalities is best to assess the abnormality further?

    a. Ultrasound abdomen

    b. MRCP

    c. No further imaging required

    d. ERCP

    e. Triple-phase CT scan of the abdomen

After further analgesia and antiemetics in the department, he feels much better and would like to go home.

You review the blood tests, and they are within normal limits with a very slight rise in the ALP and ALT only.

3. Which of the following is the best management option at this stage?

    a. Advise admission under acute internal medicine team

    b. Advise admission under the general surgery team

    c. Discharge but ask the GP to refer for further investigation

    d. Discharge but review in acute internal medicine/HPB hot clinic in 1–2 days

    e. Discharge and advise no further follow-up required

☑ 1a Biliary duct dilatation

The CT slice shown above shows significant intrahepatic biliary dilatation, most likely due to obstruction at the biliary reconstruction site. This may be due to stricture or adhesions, or recurrence of the hydatid disease. Once biliary duct dilatation is identified, it is important to establish which part of the system is dilated: intrahepatic, extrahepatic or both. Intrahepatic dilatation alone could be seen in intrahepatic cholangiocarcinoma, recurrent cholangitis or biliary necrosis; extrahepatic dilatation alone could be seen in early choledocholithiasis, pregnancy or chronic opioid use. Both intra- and extrahepatic dilatation are seen in pancreatic or ampulla mass, gallstones, pancreatitis, external compression of the common bile duct (for example, Mirizzi syndrome) and ascending cholangitis. The hyperdensity visualised within the tract is likely a stent from previous surgery and not a biliary stone (which are not well visualised on CT imaging), there is no cystic structure in the liver suggestive of recurrence of hydatid disease, and the large bowel is not visualised and therefore obstruction is unlikely, and though CT is not the most sensitive investigation for suspected gastric adenocarcinoma, there is no focal wall thickening or suggestion of a mass.

☑ 2b MRCP

The biliary tree is not visualised well on CT scan but given the dilatation of the biliary tract, this patient warrants further imaging. In the context of acute abdominal pain in a patient with history of hepatectomy, this presentation would warrant an urgent MRCP during daytime hours in order to visualise the structures of the hepatopancreatobiliary system in greater detail and determine the cause of this biliary obstruction. Though ultrasound is the most common first line investigation for suspected biliary pathology, given this patient's previous surgery it would be prudent to opt for MRCP as the next imaging modality to assess the operative site. MRCP produces high-quality images that allow diagnosis of pancreaticobiliary tree pathology without the associated risks of ERCP. Patients must be fasted for 4 hours to reduce secretions, reduce bowel peristalsis and promote gallbladder distension. All protocols are heavily T2-weighted sequences.

☑ 3d Discharge but review in acute internal medicine/HPB hot clinic in 1–2 days

Hospital admission is not needed as this patient is stable, is not displaying signs of sepsis and is not jaundiced. He has also had symptomatic improvement after treatment in the department. Therefore, it would be appropriate to discharge if you are able to arrange appropriate urgent follow-up, for example via the use of a hot clinic would be the most suitable option. If the patient was septic, had ongoing pain despite analgesia or there was evidence of cholangitis, this would be an indication for admission. In the majority of UK hospitals the admitting team for gallbladder disease is the general surgery team;

however, in some institutions, particularly large teaching hospitals, HPB gastroenterologists may admit. It is important to familiarise yourself with local procedures where you are working. If discharging from the ED, ensure that the patient has adequate analgesia to take home and provide safety net advice regarding when to return, for example, fever, rigor, jaundice, intractable pain. GP follow-up and/or referral is likely to take too long as this patient is symptomatic and therefore urgent investigation is required, and an ambulatory hot clinic would be an ideal option for this patient whereby repeat blood tests and MRCP could be coordinated.

KEY LEARNING POINTS

- Think about causes of any cylindrical structure obstruction under the headings of in the lumen, in the wall and extrinsic lesions.
- MRCP remains the gold standard for imaging the biliary tree and does not cause pancreatitis which might be seen post-ERCP.
- When thinking about further investigation, consider ambulating patients into speciality clinics to better manage flow and reduced unnecessary admissions. Local knowledge of services is key.

Seizure and leg trauma

A 30-year-old man is brought to the emergency department by ambulance after a witnessed tonic-clonic seizure that terminated prior to ambulance crew arrival. It is difficult to obtain much more history, but the crew inform you the man had been out drinking with friends the night before. He denies any other previous seizures, but his past medical history includes a complex right tibia-fibula fracture with non-union. He has recently stopped taking gabapentin.

Initial observations are recorded as HR 106, BP 118/72, SpO$_2$ 98% on room air, RR 24, temperature 37.8°C (100.0°F), GCS 15/15. On examination, he is distressed and agitated, complaining of severe pain in his left shoulder and in the right hip. Compliance with examination is poor despite analgesia and use of Entonox.

1. Which of the following is an UNLIKELY cause of seizure in this case?
    a. Gabapentin withdrawal
    b. Infection
    c. Hypoglycaemia
    d. Head injury
    e. Pain

The patient declines blood tests and continues to be challenging. You are unable to perform any further clinical examination.

Plain radiographs are requested of the right hip and left shoulder, but the patient only allows the radiographers to do a supine pelvic radiograph due to significant pain on movement.

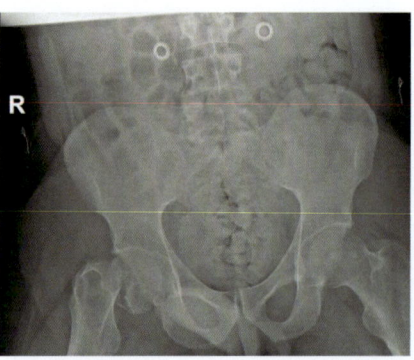

DOI: 10.1201/9781003461456-51

2. Based on the findings, which of the following is the next best management?

    a. Defer radiographs of the shoulder and refer to acute internal medicine for seizure management

    b. Trauma call, primary survey, consider CT polytrauma

    c. Request CT abdomen & pelvis with contrast only

    d. Refer to orthopaedics and ask them to perform a secondary survey

    e. Perform eFAST point-of-care ultrasound scan

3. Which blood vessel contributes the majority of the blood supply to the femoral head?

    a. Medial circumflex artery

    b. Artery to the head of the femur

    c. Lateral circumflex artery

    d. Superior gluteal artery

    e. Inferior gluteal artery

☑ 1e Pain

When patients present with a first seizure episode it is important to consider and exclude all potential reversible causes, of which there are a multitude. In this case, clues could include recent cessation of gabapentin, low-grade temperature on arrival suggestive of infection and alcohol consumption, which can cause hypoglycaemia and potential head injury if he had been intoxicated. Other conditions can cause generalised or focal CNS insult, which can reduce seizure threshold, for example electrolyte abnormalities (hyper or hyponatraemia, hypercalcaemia), metabolic disturbances (uraemia), hypoxia, intoxication, drug withdrawal (in particular alcohol, barbiturates, benzodiazepines), intracranial haemorrhage (traumatic or atraumatic) and CNS infection. Pain can lead to reflex anoxic episodes that are spontaneously reversing brief episodes of asystole due to increased vagal responsiveness, but these are non-epileptiform events.

☑ 2b Trauma call, primary survey, consider CT polytrauma

The AP pelvis radiograph shows a right sided intracapsular neck of femur (NOF) fracture. One would expect for a young patient to have sustained a fractured NOF there must have been significant force involved, and it is essential to exclude further trauma and not focus on a distracting injury, which can be difficult when the patient is doing so. A trauma call gets all the right people in the right place quickly for a primary survey before any further investigations are arranged. In UK hospitals, the trauma team will usually consist of a leader, typically an emergency medicine registrar or consultant, primary survey doctor, typically emergency medicine or general surgery doctor, anaesthetist and/or intensive care doctor, senior orthopaedic and general surgeons, nursing staff, scribe and runner(s). Trusts typically have a standardised list of scenarios when a trauma call should be activated. A full trauma 'pan-scan' (CT head, neck, chest, abdomen & pelvis) would be the next step to exclude any occult injury. In this patient, the CT identified three thoracic vertebral fractures that could have otherwise been missed as the patient reported no back pain. It also showed a fracture-dislocation of the left gleno-humeral joint. Pain management is highly important, particularly as a distressed patient can add to the stress of a trauma call. Fascia-iliaca block is the gold standard for a fractured NOF, but performing this should not delay excluding any other major traumatic injuries.

☑ 3a Medial circumflex artery

The arterial supply to the hip joint is largely via the medial and lateral circumflex femoral arteries – branches of the profunda femoris artery (deep femoral artery). They anastomose at the base of the femoral neck to form a ring, from which smaller arteries arise to supply the hip joint itself. The medial circumflex femoral artery is responsible for the majority of the arterial supply. In contrast, the lateral circumflex femoral artery has to penetrate through the thick iliofemoral ligament. Damage to the medial circumflex femoral artery can result in avascular necrosis of the femoral head. The artery to head of femur and the superior/inferior gluteal arteries all provide some additional supply. Other joints that are most at risk of avascular necrosis are the humeral head, patella and talus.

KEY LEARNING POINTS

- Think widely but in a systematic manner when considering causes of seizures – the box (brain), the pump (cardiac), the wiring (nerves and vascular), medications including lack of, and electrolytes. Don't forget glucose too!
- In cases of unexpected injury in a young patient or high kinetic energy mechanisms, remember that putting out a trauma call will bring the relevant senior expertise to the patient and provides a standardised assessment and management protocol.
- The blood supply to the femoral head is supplied by the cruciate anastomosis but compromised in intracapsular fractures meaning that hemiarthroplasty or total hip replacement is often needed.

CASE 52

Seizures in an international student

A 22-year-old man, who is an international university student from India, presents to the emergency department (ED) after a 'blackout'. His girlfriend describes witnessing him become rigid and then have all over body shaking with loss of consciousness lasting around 3 minutes. He was drowsy for around 30 minutes after this episode, and it was noted that he had bitten his tongue. He has been otherwise well in preceding days with no prodromal illness. He denies headache, visual disturbance and peripheral weakness or sensory change. He has no past medical history and has never experienced this before.

Initial observations are within normal limits, he is afebrile and GCS 15/15. Capillary blood glucose is normal. He looks generally well. Cranial nerve and peripheral nervous system, including gait, examinations do not detect any abnormality.

1. Which investigation is NOT routinely recommended in the ED for this presentation?
   a. ECG
   b. Venous blood gas (VBG), FBC, U&E, LFT, CRP, bone profile & magnesium
   c. CT head
   d. Urine dip
   e. Blood glucose testing

On review of the ED investigations, the VBG is normal and the ECG shows normal sinus rhythm.

Chest radiograph shows clear lung fields.

Blood results reveal WCC 14, with neutrophils 11, CRP and remaining biochemistry results are within normal limits.

A CT head is performed following a further witnessed seizure episode in the department. This shows a *small 3 mm focus of high density in keeping with blood product and associated with oedema is present in the right posterior high convexity.*

The patient is admitted under the acute internal medicine team and subsequently undergoes an MRI brain with contrast for further characterisation.

DOI: 10.1201/9781003461456-52

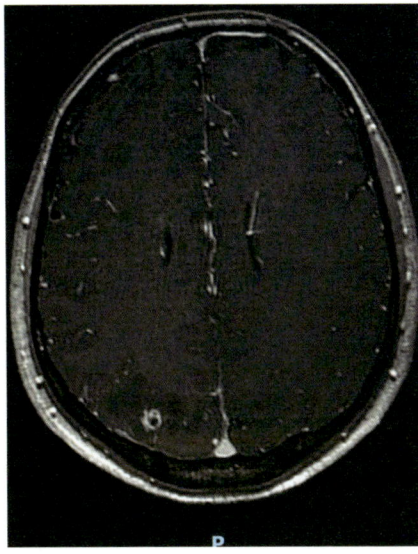

2. Which of the following is the best description of what this image shows?

    a. Glioblastoma multiforme

    b. Cerebral ring-enhancing lesion

    c. Parietal arteriovenous malformation (AVM)

    d. Meningioma

    e. Cortical ribboning indicative of CJD

3. Based on the MRI imaging, which of the following initial investigations would be your next step to confirm the suspected diagnosis?

    a. Surgical brain biopsy

    b. Electroencephalogram (EEG)

    c. Lumbar puncture and serology for TB and neurocysticerosis

    d. Anti-NMDA receptor antibodies

    e. High-resolution CT chest

☑ 1c CT head

The likely diagnosis here is a first seizure, which sounds like it was tonic-clonic in nature. Indications for CT head in the ED include recurrent seizures or status epilepticus, focal neurological deficit, reduced GCS, headache, head injury, pyrexia, immunosuppression, history of cancer, BP >180/120, anticoagulation. Based on these indications, our patient does not meet the criteria for CT head but should have the other investigations to exclude reversible causes of seizure. Hypoglycaemia is already excluded, blood work will evaluate for electrolyte abnormalities and inflammatory markers, urine dip and chest radiograph also look for infection and ECG evaluates for cardiac abnormalities that may predispose to syncope. If these results were normal, this patient could be discharged with safety net advice, advice to stop driving and alert the appropriate driving licensing authority, and referral to first-fit clinic for follow-up and further investigation including imaging.

☑ 2b Cerebral ring-enhancing lesion

There is a solitary right parietal bilobed ring-enhancing lesion associated with calcification. The solitary nature of the lesion is more consistent for tuberculosis although neurocysticercosis remains a differential with this patient's background. The lesion could represent a solitary metastasis but does not have features of glioblastoma, which is often seen with an irregular border and enhancements with variable centres. There is no evidence of an AVM; fast flow generates flow voids on T2 images in AVMs and possible haemorrhage surrounding this along with adjacent oedema. Cortical ribboning is a sensitive feature of MR flair imaging when investigating for CJD, which is high signal on diffusion-weighted imaging in the white matter. These changes are generally patchy but involve more than one cortical region. The clinical features often correlate with the site of cortical signal change. Note that the presentation in this case is not consistent with CJD, and there is no cortical ribboning.

☑ 3c Lumbar puncture and serology for TB and neurocysticerosis

Given that the suspected diagnosis is cerebral TB or neurocysticerosis based on the ring-enhancing lesion that is seen on the MRI head, a lumbar puncture for microscopy and culture, cysticercosis serology and tuberculosis PCR and culture would be the most useful investigation. High-resolution CT chest is unlikely to be useful in the absence of constitutional or respiratory symptoms of tuberculosis but may be considered if the lumbar puncture is positive. An EEG is not required as the seizure history is convincing and it is unlikely to provide further diagnostic information in this case. Anti-NMDA receptor antibodies would be useful if there was an indication of autoimmune encephalitis. Surgical brain biopsy is the final possible investigation if all others do not provide a diagnosis. This patient went on to have a lumbar puncture with CSF serology testing for cysticercosis returning as positive. He has since commenced treatment and was followed up by the infectious diseases team. Neurocysticerosis occurs as a result of infection with *Taenia solium* tapeworm. Larvae can develop in many organs, including skin, eyes, muscle and CNS. Neurocysticerosis occurs when cysts form in the brain and is estimated as the cause of 30% of epilepsy in countries where *T. solium* is endemic.

KEY LEARNING POINTS

- CT head scans are not currently routinely recommended for patients presenting with a first seizure. However, clinical judgement should be applied to each patient and imaging should be performed in high-risk patients or where there is a strong suspicion of an underlying lesion.
- MRI provides highly detailed imaging of cerebral structures, which can be further enhanced with gadolinium.
- Neurocysticerosis is caused by the tapeworm *Taenia solium*, which can be deposited in many organs where cysts can remain dormant for many years. Diagnosis may be made by direct biopsy, serology or PCR testing.

Sepsis

A 35-year-old man presents to the emergency department (ED) complaining of a 3-week history of non-bloody diarrhoea and intermittent fevers. On further questioning, he informs you he has been suffering with intermittent diarrhoea over the last few months. His symptoms have worsened in the last 48 hours with rigors and pre-syncopal symptoms on arrival to the ED. He has no nausea or vomiting, no cough or shortness of breath, no urinary frequency or urgency. There is no travel history, and he denies recreational drug use.

Initial observations are recorded as HR 112, BP 122/58, SpO$_2$ 100% on room air, RR 21, temperature 39.4°C (102.9°F). On examination, he looks unwell, is sweaty and clammy, with dry mucous membranes. His abdomen is soft with generalised tenderness.

A venous blood gas (VBG) is performed and reveals pH 7.42, pCO$_2$ 4.2, HCO$_3^-$ 20.7, BE –3.7, Lactate 5.7, Na$^+$ 134, K$^+$ 3.2, Cr 136, urea 4.1, glucose 4.2.

He is fluid resuscitated with 2 L of IV crystalloid fluid over 1 hour.

A CT abdomen & pelvis with contrast is performed once physiologically stable.

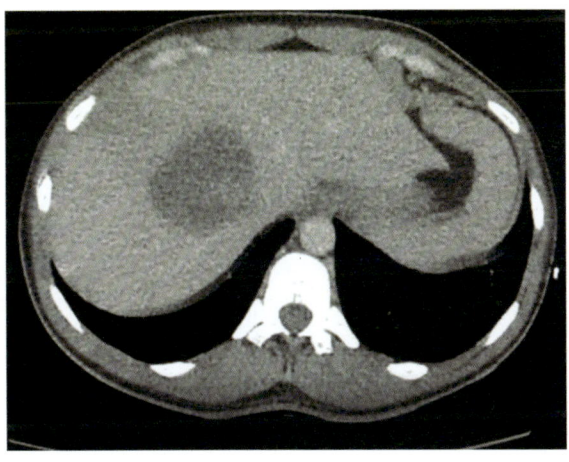

DOI: 10.1201/9781003461456-53

1. Which of the following diagnoses is suggested by the CT abdomen & pelvis?

    a. Simple hepatic cyst

    b. Liver metastases with colonic primary

    c. Acute appendicitis

    d. Right basal pneumonia

    e. Pyogenic liver abscess

The patient's blood pressure is labile despite further fluid resuscitation and fails to respond to fluid boluses. Boluses of metaraminol are now required and therefore you insert an arterial line and commence a noradrenaline infusion.

You review the laboratory blood results and note Hb 112, WCC 5.01, CRP 322, creatinine 149, eGFR 48, ALP 193, ALT 76, albumin 35, bilirubin 26, Troponin T 40.

The patient is reviewed by the intensive care unit registrar who performs a point-of-care echocardiogram, which shows:

1. Mildly dilated globally hypokinetic LV with mild LV impairment
2. Moderately dilated RV but good function but longitudinal and radial function
3. Trace MR and mild TR

You review the ECG again.

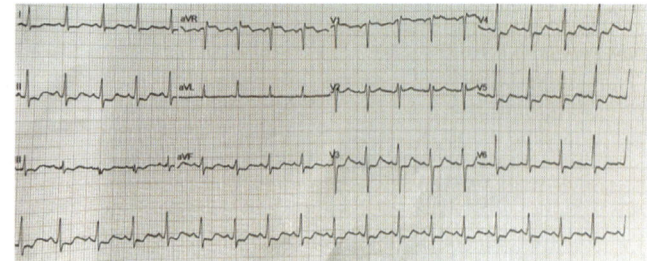 

2. Which of the following best accounts for the ECG appearances in this case?

    a. Hypertrophic obstructive cardiomyopathy

    b. Non-ST elevation myocardial infarction

    c. Cocaine related cardiomyopathy

    d. Septic cardiomyopathy

    e. Cardiogenic shock

3. Which of the following is the most likely underlying condition in this patient that led to the complication seen on the CT?

    a. Diabetes mellitus

    b. Inflammatory bowel disease or chronic appendicitis

    c. NSAID-induced gastritis

    d. Acute cholecystitis

    e. Community-acquired pneumonia

☑ 1e Pyogenic liver abscess

The CT shows a large area of low attenuation centrally in the liver (measuring approximately 7 cm x 6 cm x 6 cm), which most likely represents an abscess. Incidental hepatic cysts are almost always asymptomatic and are generally seen as homogeneous hypoattenuation with imperceptible walls and do not enhance with contrast. They may be found anywhere in the liver but have a predilection for the right lobe. Liver metastases are most commonly be seen as multiple lesions. The CT does show an inflammatory process around the right iliac fossa with fat stranding and a trace of free pelvic fluid, which could be suggestive of acute appendicitis. However, the clinical picture of a prolonged history with swinging fevers, rigors and sepsis are more suggestive of an abscess than acute appendicitis. Chronic inflammation of the appendix can occur, which typically presents as recurrent or chronic lower abdominal pain associated with fever; diarrhoea and sepsis are unlikely symptoms in these cases. Terminal ileitis alone would not generally lead to a patient being so clinically unwell. There are no changes within the right lung base suggestive of consolidation.

☑ 2d Septic cardiomyopathy

Sepsis-induced cardiomyopathy is a feature of severe sepsis and septic shock which results in a reversible myocardial depression and impaired contractility due to ventricular dilatation, leading to reduced ejection fracture despite maintained stroke volume. This is the most likely cause given the global picture of septic shock. Noradrenaline leads to increased systemic vascular resistance and reduced cardiac output, which can 'unmask' septic cardiomyopathy. It typically resolves within 7 days in survivors. Type 2 myocardial infarction can occur secondary to ischaemia due to increased oxygen demand or decreased supply, for example, secondary to anaemia, arrhythmia or hypotension. However, you would still expect symptoms of MI, which are not present in this case, and a more dramatic increase in Troponin T. Cocaine related cardiomyopathy requires high level chronic use of cocaine and the patient denies any previous use. It typically leads to a dilated cardiomyopathy. He did not have any features suggestive of cardiogenic shock (for example, acute shortness of breath or signs of fluid overload). ECG features of hypertrophic obstructive cardiomyopathy (HOCM) are left ventricular hypertrophy with deep and narrow Q waves in lateral and/or inferior leads; echo shows marked left ventricular hypertrophy with non-dilated ventricles.

☑ 3b Inflammatory bowel disease or chronic appendicitis

In developed countries, three quarters of hepatic abscesses are pyogenic in origin. Most of these are secondary to infection elsewhere in the body via haematogenous or biliary spread. A major risk factor is underlying immunosuppression, for example due to diabetes, HIV, malignancy, renal failure or elderly. Depending on the immune status of the patient and the underlying organism, hepatic abscesses can present acutely or with grumbling vague signs. Of the presented options; inflammatory bowel disease, cholecystitis, appendicitis are all potential causes of liver abscesses, and diabetes is a risk factor. NSAID-induced gastritis by itself is not commonly associated with liver abscesses. Looking at the overall history and the CT findings of right iliac fossa and pelvic inflammation alongside the liver lesion, the most likely underlying cause of the abscess in this patient is inflammatory bowel disease or chronic appendicitis. Non-pyogenic abscesses are classified as amoebic or fungal, caused by *Entamoeba histolytica* and most often *Candida* species, respectively.

KEY LEARNING POINTS

- Liver abscesses may present insidiously with swinging fevers and RUQ pain over months. Haematogenous seeding is the most common cause.
- On CT, simple hepatic cysts have well defined walls with no enhancement with contrast compared to a liver abscess or metastatic deposit.
- Septic cardiomyopathy may be seen in critically unwell patient with characteristic ECG findings. In patients who survive, the changes may be reversible with significant myocardial recovery.

CASE 54

Severe respiratory distress

A 48-year-old woman is brought in by ambulance to the emergency department (ED) in severe respiratory distress. She is known to have had severe asthma since childhood and is currently on a weaning dose of steroids. She has recently tested positive for COVID-19. On arrival, she is immediately transferred to the resuscitation room and an arrest call (code blue) is made to alert appropriate specialty teams.

You perform an initial assessment immediately on transfer:

1. Airway: maintaining own airway, no stridor or other added sounds
2. Breathing: sitting forward in the tripod position, unable to complete sentences, SpO_2 88% on 15 L oxygen via non-rebreathe mask, RR 40, poor air entry bilaterally, no audible wheeze noted
3. Circulation: peripheries are cool and shut down, CRT 3 seconds centrally, HR 132, BP 142/77
4. Disability: GCS 15/15, CBG 7.7
5. Exposure: appears to be tiring

1. Which one of the following features would suggest a life-threatening asthma exacerbation?

    a. FEV_1 of 30–50% best or predicted

    b. Inability to complete full sentences

    c. HR >110 bpm

    d. RR >25/min

    e. $PaCO_2$ >6 kPa (45 mmHg)

Despite maximal medical management with back-to-back salbutamol and ipratropium nebulisers, IV magnesium sulphate and IV aminophylline, there is little improvement in her clinical picture. The acute internal medicine, anaesthetic and intensive care unit teams are all in attendance and it is agreed that she needs emergency intubation.

Once intubated, she is ventilated using the anaesthetic machine in the resuscitation bay using the following settings: volume-controlled ventilation (VCV), FiO_2 0.8, TV 200 mL, RR 12, I:E 1:5, PEEP 10 cmH_2O.

However, after approximately 30 minutes, there is an abrupt rise in peak airway pressures and reduction in tidal volume with associated desaturation to SpO_2 75% on FiO_2 1.0, with tachycardia of 149 and hypotension of 85/50.

DOI: 10.1201/9781003461456-54

2. Which of the following is the most likely complication to have occurred?

    a. Displacement of the endotracheal tube

    b. Obstruction of the endotracheal tube secondary to mucous plugging

    c. Endotracheal tube cuff leak

    d. Salbutamol toxicity

    e. Tension pneumothorax

Once stabilised, a portable chest radiograph is performed.

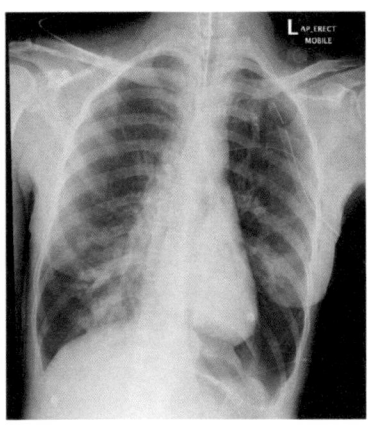

3. How would you best describe the findings of the chest radiograph?

    a. This is a PA chest radiograph. There is the presence of right lower lobe consolidation. Clinical correlation is advised

    b. This is a mobile AP film. There is the presence of bilateral lower zone consolidation suggestive of acute pneumonia

    c. This is a mobile AP film. There is the presence of collapse behind the left ventricle (LV) (sail-sign) suggestive of either infection or a posterior mediastinal mass. Clinical correlation is advised

    d. This is a mobile AP film. There is the presence of an endotracheal tube with the tip approximately 2.5 cm below the medial clavicles. There is right basal consolidation, which may correspond to aspiration. On the left there is the presence of two intercostal drains and a moderate residual pneumothorax. Note is made of a fine bore NG tube appearing to bisect the carina and pass through the diaphragm

    e. This is a mobile PA film. There is the presence of an endotracheal tube passing into the right main bronchus causing lower lobe collapse. On the left, note is made of two intercostal drains with one pointing towards the apex of the lung. There is a wide bore NG tube, which appears to be passed in the fundus of the stomach

☑ 1e PaCO$_2$ > 6 kPa (45 mmHg)

Management of acute asthma in the ED is time-critical and requires rapid assessment to determine severity and initiation of appropriate treatment. In the initial assessment, you are determining if moderate, severe or life-threatening features are present. A review of the patient should be performed along with measurement of peak-expiratory flow rate (PEFR) if possible, oxygen saturations, respiratory rate and heart rate and the chest should be auscultated. Life-threatening asthma is indicated by PEFR <33% of best or predicted, SpO$_2$ <92%, silent chest and poor respiratory effort, hypotension, arrhythmia, exhaustion or altered consciousness. Any one of these life-threatening features means the patient should be treated as such, with immediate administration of nebulised bronchodilator therapy, supplemental oxygen as necessary and steroids. Arterial blood gas analysis should then be performed, looking for hypoxia (PaO$_2$ <8 kPa), 'normal' (4.5–6.0 kPa) or raised (> 6.0 kPa) PaCO$_2$ and acidaemia. Always consider when you need to call for senior help and to alert intensive care specialists of the unwell patient.

☑ 2e Tension pneumothorax

The abrupt change of settings on the ventilator, along with haemodynamic instability and decreased breath sounds, makes the diagnosis of a tension pneumothorax the most likely of the provided options. Bronchospasm in asthma leads to increased airway resistance, which is worsened by airway inflammation and mucous that can occur in infective exacerbations. There are two main issues with intermittent positive pressure ventilation due to this increased airway resistance: firstly, higher pressures are required to drive the gases to achieve a tidal volume and secondly, air trapping and hyperinflation can occur due to reduced expiratory flow. This leads to the risk of barotrauma and pneumothorax as a consequence, and also haemodynamic instability due to increased intrathoracic pressure. There are a number of strategies that can reduce the risks associated with mechanical ventilation in patients with asthma. Firstly, reduce resistance by using the largest endotracheal tube and removing as much dead space as possible in the circuit. Secondly, use volume-controlled mode with constant flow with small protective tidal volumes (5–7 mL/kg), a slow respiratory rate, long expiratory time (inspiratory/expiratory ratio 1:3 or 1:4), and minimal PEEP. However, this patient did not tolerate a reduced PEEP and therefore it was maintained at 10 cmH$_2$O. Ensure to keep the plateau pressure below 25 cmH20 to prevent dynamic hyperinflation. Use of neuromuscular blockade (for example, rocuronium) can be used if necessary to facilitate synchronicity with the ventilator. The main learning point in this case is that just because a patient with asthma has been intubated, this is not the end of the story.

☑ **3d This is a mobile AP film. There is the presence of an endotracheal tube with the tip approximately 2.5 cm below the medial clavicles. There is right basal consolidation, which may correspond to aspiration. On the left there is the presence of two intercostal drains and a moderate residual pneumothorax. Note is made of a fine bore NG tube appearing to bisect the carina and pass through the diaphragm**

Chest radiographs are not only useful for assessing lung pathology but can also be used for reviewing tubes and lines that may have been inserted into critically unwell patients. Always remember to use a systematic approach to reviewing chest radiographs to ensure no abnormalities are missed. The simplest one is ABCDE, where A = airway (trachea), B = breathing (lung fields and pleura), C = circulation (heart and great vessels), D = diaphragm and E = everything else. Using this system, we can see that this patient has been intubated. Following the tube down, we can see the tip lying about 2.5 cm below the medial end of the clavicles; whilst acceptable here, it might be advanced further slightly especially if the patient is to be transferred to ITU or elsewhere, to prevent it falling out. Considering the right lung first, there is lower lobe consolidation, which might be a primary infective process or indeed aspiration pneumonia. The left side is complex; there are two intercostal drains with one pointing towards the lung apex. Following the pleural edge down to the bottom of the lung, we can see the presence of a sizeable residual pneumothorax. This would be in keeping with a large air leak that is still not fully drained – one might need to upsize the smaller of the two intercostal drains. The heart and mediastinum reassuringly are still in the midline, showing that we do not have any radiological suggestion of tension pneumothorax. Looking at the diaphragm, we can see a fine bore NG tube passing below and it can be traced upwards to the upper oesophagus without issue. Lastly, there are ECG leads, the pilot balloon of the endotracheal tube over the left lung apex and a nebuliser venturi chamber just adjacent to it.

Although seemingly straightforward, the humble chest radiograph can provide a huge amount of information if interpreted in a systematic and methodical manner. Overall, this radiograph illustrates a very unwell patient who has suffered from significant barotrauma and a very large resultant air-leak needing the placement of not one, but two intercostal drains. Onward management will be tricky, and options might include consideration of extra-corporeal membrane oxygenation (ECMO) if ventilation and oxygenation remain problematic. The objective of this treatment is to mitigate ventilator-induced lung injury and provide adequate time for the inflammatory processes in the lungs to diminish. This patient was accepted for ECMO and subsequently did well.

KEY LEARNING POINTS

- Asthmatic patients can present in extremis and deteriorate rapidly despite medical management; it is important to get senior help and the ICU team involved early.
- Asthmatic patients requiring mechanical ventilation are at risk due to barotrauma and dynamic hyperinflation.
- The chest radiograph remains a valuable tool in the management of acutely unwell patients if interpreted in a systematic and methodical manner.

CASE 55

Short of breath at rest

A 74-year-old man presents to the emergency department (ED) having been brought in by ambulance. He has been holidaying for the last 2 weeks on the UK south coast, enjoying strolls by the beach and visiting friends. He was on his way back home via train and had been sitting for about 2 and a half hours. Whilst on the train, he started to become very short of breath and feel tremulous. The ambulance service was called and noted his saturations to be transiently as low as 88%. Past medical history includes hypertension for which he takes amlodipine and atenolol. He mentions that he was seen in his local hospital one month ago and was told he had a 'blocked artery in the heart'. Further details are vague.

Initial observations are recorded as HR 66, BP 153/70, SpO$_2$ 94% on room air, RR 17, temperature 36.6°C (97.9°F). On examination, you note a 4/6 systolic murmur audible throughout the precordium. Auscultation of the chest reveals fine inspiratory crepitations worse on the right than the left. Calves are soft, but you note the presence of pitting oedema bilaterally up to the knees.

An ECG is performed.

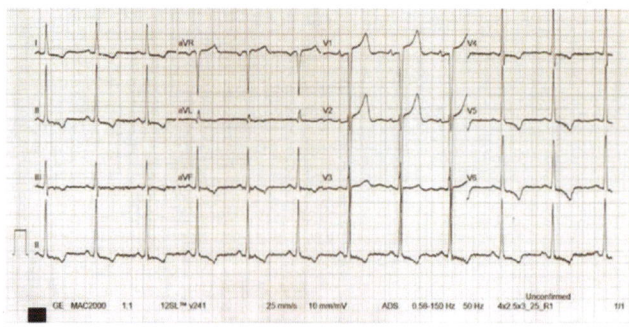

1. Which of the following features are present on the ECG?
   a. Sinus tachycardia
   b. S1Q3T3 pattern
   c. Left ventricular hypertrophy (LVH) with strain pattern
   d. Left bundle branch block
   e. Pathological Q waves

You request a standard blood set of FBC, U&E, coagulation profile and CRP.

DOI: 10.1201/9781003461456-55

2. Which of the following is the best additional management steps for this man in the ED based on the history and examination findings?

    a. Move to the resuscitation room and consider thrombolysis

    b. Troponin T, calculate Wells score, chest radiograph, serial ECGs, refer to acute internal medicine

    c. D-dimer and ambulate for next day V/Q scan

    d. Three sets of blood cultures, and refer to infectious diseases

    e. Chest radiograph, and physiotherapy assessment as he has a train to catch home

As part of the work-up in the department, a point-of-care echocardiogram is performed. The parasternal long axis (PLAX) view is shown.

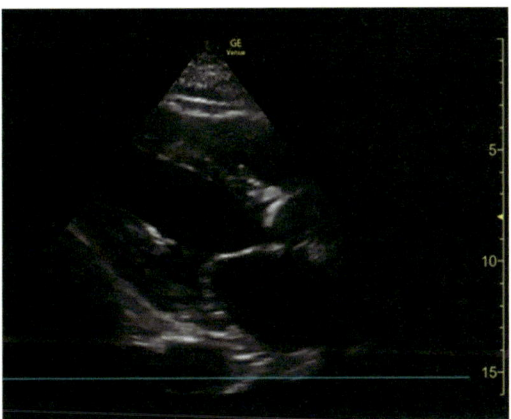

3. Which of the following is the best description of what is seen?

    a. Aortic stenosis

    b. Pulmonary stenosis

    c. Ischaemic cardiomyopathy

    d. Pulmonary embolus

    e. Mitral valve stenosis

☑   1c Left ventricular hypertrophy with strain pattern

This ECG shows sinus rhythm (but not tachycardia), LVH with strain and the presence of U waves. When assessing any ECG, remember to start with the basics: patient details, date and time, lead placement, speed (25 mm/s) and amplitude (10 mm/mV). Then review the trace itself by checking that there is a P wave in front of each QRS complex, indicating sinus rhythm. Then review the P wave morphology (normal, p-pulmonale, p-mitrale) and its distance to the QRS complex; the PR interval is normally 3–5 small squares. On this ECG, we can clearly see sinus rhythm. Moving on to the QRS complex, assess the height and width of the complexes. The striking abnormality on this trace is the very tall complexes. This can be normal in slim patients, but in this context represents LVH. The Sokolov–Lyon criteria for LVH is S wave depth in V1 + tallest R wave height in V5 or V6 is >35 mm. The apparent ST elevation in V1–3 is proportional to the very deep S waves in these leads and is known as 'appropriate discordance'. Looking next at the T waves, there is widespread inversion (V4–6, II, III, aVF). Coupled with the LVH this is known as a 'strain pattern'. Lastly, if you look carefully after the T waves, you can see prominent U waves especially in V1–3.

☑   2b Troponin T, calculate Wells score, chest radiograph, serial ECGs, refer to acute internal medicine

The most important aspect is to exclude an acute coronary syndrome (ACS) event by sending Troponin T and monitoring serial ECGs. In the presence of suspected aortic stenosis (shortness of breath, systolic murmur and signs of heart failure), this patient has significant risks for coronary artery disease and thus ACS. The processes that cause long-term calcification of the aortic valve can also result in the atherosclerosis of the coronary arteries. The presence of the bibasal crepitations and peripheral oedema suggests clinical heart failure too. The transient low saturations could point to either a PE or transient pulmonary oedema, which is more likely in his case. Should further history and examination elicit concern for a PE, calculate the Wells score before sending a D-dimer. This patient is high risk for either ACS or sudden decompensation from his suspected severe aortic stenosis and will need admission under the acute internal medicine team. In this patient, the diagnosis of AS was confirmed on formal echocardiography; serial Troponins were stable at around 32.

☑   3a Aortic stenosis

The correct answer is aortic stenosis. The PLAX is the 'go-to' initial view when looking at the heart and gives excellent views of the left side of the heart. Firstly, orientate the image in your mind. The apex of the heart is at the top left of the image. The large cavity in the centre is the LV with the mitral valve. To the bottom right, we can see the left atrium and just above this we can visualise the left ventricular outflow tract (LVOT) and the aortic valve. The right ventricle is at the top of the image in the centre. The first abnormality is the bright, white, echogenic aortic valve (AV). Looking at the AV, you will note that it is barely opening. No cusp motion and decrease in the maximal cusp separation are echocardiographic features of severe AS. The LV wall appears thickened too, suggestive of hypertrophy. Note that the mitral valve, although moving, appears to be slightly 'lazy', raising the suspicion of mitral regurgitation too. These findings would correlate to the clinical findings and the ECG.

KEY LEARNING POINTS

- A careful history, clinical examination and simple investigations are usually sufficient to make a preliminary diagnosis in cases of new cardiac murmurs.
- ECG findings of left ventricular hypertrophy include tall QRS complexes, ST-depression and T-wave inversion.
- Point-of-care echocardiography skills can be readily acquired to augment diagnosis particularly in cases of left-sided valvular dysfunction (MV, AV, stenosis or regurgitation).

Shortness of breath and palpitations

A 78-year-old man was advised to attend the nearest emergency department by his GP. He has been suffering from increasing shortness of breath, worse upon walking uphill, with paroxysmal nocturnal dyspnoea for the last 2 months. His GP had arranged some blood tests and an outpatient ECG.

His past medical history includes a previous STEMI, hypertension,type 2 diabetes mellitus, hypercholesterolaemia, depression and anxiety.

Initial observations are recorded as HR 75, BP 139/88, SpO$_2$ 97% on room air, RR 17, temperature 36.8°C (98.4°F). On examination, the patient appears well and can maintain a conversation without getting out of breath. Heart sounds appear to be normal, JVP is not elevated, the chest is clear and there is minimal peripheral oedema.

An ECG is performed.

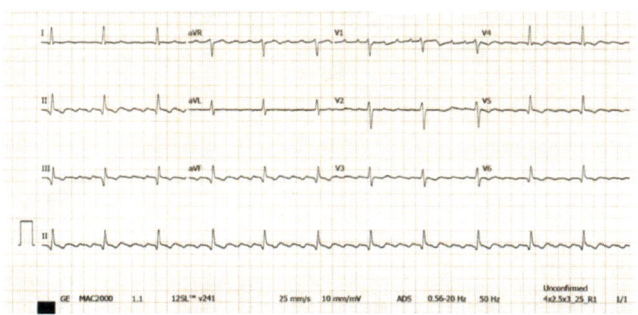 

1. Which of the following is the most likely diagnosis?

    a. Atrial fibrillation

    b. Atrial flutter

    c. Junctional rhythm

    d. Atrioventricular node re-entrant tachycardia

    e. Ventricular fibrillation

DOI: 10.1201/9781003461456-56

Bloods are drawn and you review the venous blood gas (VBG) result.

POCT VENOUS BLOOD GAS

Component			
Ref Range & Units	4d ago		
Source	Venous	**Total Haemoglobin**	138
pH	7.386	g/l	
Carbon Dioxide Partial Pressure	7.37^	**Deoxyhaemoglobin**	72.4^
kPa		%	
Comment: Value above reference range		Comment: Value above reference range	
Oxygen Partial Pressure	2.57ᵥ	**Oxyhaemoglobin**	25.4ᵥ
kPa		%	
Comment: Value below reference range		Comment: Value below reference range	
Potassium	4.1	**Saturated Oxygen**	26.0ᵥ
mmol/L		%	
Sodium	147	Comment: Value below reference range	
mmol/L		**Carboxyhaemoglobin**	1.1
Ionised Calcium	1.24	%	
mmol/L		**Methaemoglobin**	1.1
Chloride	107^	%	
mmol/L		**Fraction of Inspired Oxygen**	21.0
Comment: Value above reference range		%	
Glucose	4.7	**Standard Base Excess**	8.1
mmol/L		mmol/L	
Lactate	0.8	**Standard Bicarbonate**	28.5
mmol/L		mmol/L	
Urea	7.4	**Haematocrit**	42.2
mmol/L		%	
Creatinine	115.2	**Oxygen tension at 50% Saturation**	3.91
micromol/l		kPa	

2. Which of the following is the best next management step for this man?

   a.   Amiodarone 200 mg PO TDS

   b.   Metoprolol 5 mg IV over 5 minutes

   c.   Flecainide 150 mg IV over 30 minutes

   d.   Anticoagulation with LMWH or DOAC

   e.   Synchronised DC cardioversion 100 J (biphasic)

3. Which of the following are risk factors for the above rhythm on the ECG?

    a. Male gender

    b. Old age

    c. Ischaemic heart disease

    d. Endurance sports

    e. All of the above

☑ 1b Atrial flutter

The ECG shows atrial flutter with 4:1 block. Note the 'saw-tooth' baseline of flutter or 'F' waves best seen in the rhythm strip lead II interspersed at regular intervals by a QRS complex. The ventricular rate is determined by the AV conduction ratio, which may be 4:1 (HR 75 bpm), 3:1 (HR 100 bpm) or 2:1 (HR 150 bpm). If you see a rate of exactly 150 bpm, this should make you highly suspicious of atrial flutter with 2:1 block. Conversely, atrial fibrillation is diagnosed with a loss of P waves, absence of the isoelectric baseline with variable ventricular rate leading to an 'irregularly irregular' rhythm with narrow QRS, unless pre-existing bundle branch block or accessory pathway is present. If the diagnosis is not obvious, the rhythm strip is often the key to diagnosis. You can also use a blank sheet of paper to mark QRS complexes and move this across the strip to review the RR interval. Junctional rhythms arise at the level of the AV node and show the morphology of a narrow QRS complex with a rate of 60 bpm or less. There may be tiny retrograde P waves either just before or after the QRS complex. Atrioventricular node re-entrant tachycardia (AVNRT) is a form of supraventricular tachycardia (SVT). Key defining features are that they are usually regular, with narrow complexes and heart rates of >140. Ventricular fibrillation is a shockable cardiac arrest rhythm; it is seen as chaotic irregular deflections of varying amplitude with no identifiable P, QRS or T waves.

☑ 2d Anticoagulation with LMWH or DOAC

There are three main considerations in the treatment of atrial flutter: ventricular rate, reversion and maintenance of sinus rhythm and prevention of venous thromboembolism, and the management will depend on the clinical presentation. In this patient, rate control is not required. If rapid control of ventricular rate was indicated, IV beta-blocker for example, metoprolol or calcium-channel blocker, for example, verapamil is usually effective. Chemical cardioversion is quite tricky with atrial flutter but agents such as dofetilide and ibutilide (pure class III agents) are effective, but there is a risk of QT prolongation and a small incidence of torsades de pointes. Flecainide (class Ic agent) may also be effective but risk dramatic reduction in the atrial rate and risk of 1:1 AV block. Amiodarone is not very effective in this setting but may provide rate control. The greatest chance of reversion to sinus rhythm with atrial flutter is electrical DC cardioversion. This must only be attempted if there is a defined onset less than 48 hours due to potential clot formation in the left atrial appendage. In this patient, as symptoms have likely been going on for 2 months or more, the best option would be to initiate anticoagulation with LMWH or DOAC after calculating stroke (CHA_2DS_2-VASc score) and bleeding risk (HASBLED score).

☑ 3e All of the above

All answers are correct! 80% of atrial flutter occurs in male patients. Risk factors for structural heart disease, including hypertension, valvular heart disease, ischaemic heart disease, chronic obstructive pulmonary disease and older age also increase the risk of developing atrial flutter. The possibly more surprising risk factor is endurance athletics. This predisposes to both atrial flutter and fibrillation. The exact mechanism is unknown, but a large body of evidence for this comes from skiers and cyclists. Possible mechanisms are thought to be due to increased vagal tone, catecholamine storms and right atrial remodelling, which is the prime site for flutter generation. The other big risk factors are following cardiac surgery (20–30%) and the initiation of anti-arrhythmic drugs, notably flecainide (15%). Atrial flutter can also occur in individuals with no prior heart problems or patients who have other atrial arrhythmias.

KEY LEARNING POINTS

- Atrial flutter can readily be identified due to the irregular saw tooth baseline caused by F waves. The HR may give a clue to the block level, for example HR 75 = 4:1 block; HR 100 = 3:1 block; HR 150 = 2:1 block.
- Atrial flutter is quite resistant to chemical cardioversion, but DC cardioversion must only be attempted in patients who are fully anticoagulated or those whose onset is less than 48 hours, due to the high risk of embolic stroke.
- Along with traditional CV risk factors, endurance athletes are at risk of atrial flutter and fibrillation due to a variety of factors (endocrine, structural).

Slurred speech

An 82-year-old woman is brought to the emergency department by her daughter. Her daughter informs you her mother suffered a fall around a week ago. Since then, she has been 'muddled' and intermittently has had slurred speech. Currently, she is living independently and has a background of hypertension, transient ischaemic attack (4 years ago) and hyperthyroidism.

You assess her in triage and note a blood pressure of 240/140. Focused neurological examination is normal and GCS 15/15.

You request bloods including FBC, U&E, CRP, coagulation profile, 12-lead ECG and urine dip.

1. Which of the following would you also include as your initial management plan from triage?
   a. Non-contrast CT head, stream to majors
   b. CT head stroke protocol, stream to resuscitation room
   c. Non-contrast CT head, amlodipine 10 mg PO, stream to majors
   d. CT head stroke protocol, labetalol 50 mg IV, stream to majors
   e. CT head stroke protocol, labetalol 50 mg IV, stream to resuscitation room

A CT is performed, and you review the images before the radiology report is available.

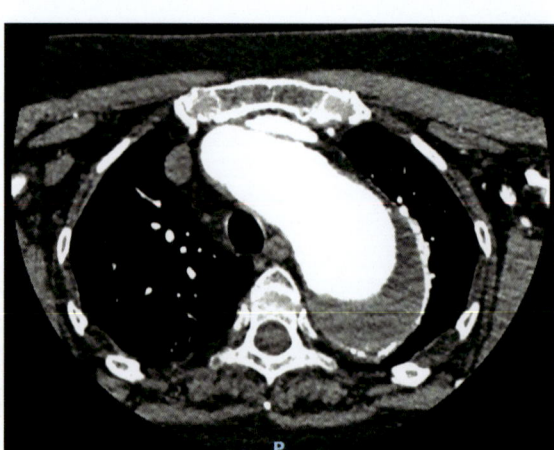

2. Which of the following best describes the most significant finding on this scan?

    a. Filling defects in the transverse venous sinus suggestive of venous sinus thrombosis

    b. Severe burden of small vessel disease with evidence of a developing right anterior cerebral artery infarct

    c. Evidence of a small amount of subarachnoid bleeding, unclear if traumatic or spontaneous in origin

    d. Right vertebral artery wall thickening with surrounding stranding indicative of mural thrombus suggestive of dissection

    e. Dilated ascending aorta, aortic arch and proximal descending aorta with filling defect suggestive of dissection

3. Based on the CT findings, which of the following is the best next management step?

    a. Ensure two large bore cannulae, labetalol 50 mg IV, refer to intensive care unit (ICU) for invasive blood pressure monitoring

    b. Group & screen, ensure two large bore cannulae, 15-minute neuro observations, refer to neurosurgeons

    c. Group & screen, ensure two large bore cannulae, labetalol 2 mg per minute IV, refer to cardiothoracic team and intensive care unit (ICU)

    d. Amlodipine 10 mg PO, refer to acute internal medicine for inpatient blood pressure monitoring

    e. Group & screen, ensure two large bore cannulae, labetalol 50 mg IV, refer to vascular surgeons

☑ 1b CT head intracranial angiogram, stream to resuscitation room

The history is deliberately vague but there are several differentials that must be considered in this type of patient that would require neuroimaging, including hypertensive intracranial haemorrhage, hypertensive encephalopathy, traumatic intracranial haemorrhage and ischaemic stroke. Given the patient has significant risk factors for possible stroke (previous TIA and profound hypertension), CT head with intracranial angiogram and discussion with the stroke or neurology team is the best option. Regarding the management of hypertension, if the patient does not show imminent signs of end organ failure, it is ideal to try and obtain imaging before lowering. If there was a significant intracranial haemorrhage with mass effect or the patient had suffered an acute ischaemic insult, lowering the blood pressure and subsequently the cerebral perfusion pressure could potentially worsen the patient outcome. Admission to a closely monitored area, such as resuscitation room, intensive or coronary care unit for IV antihypertensive treatment aiming to lower the blood pressure within minutes to 1 hour, targeting 160/100 mmHg. With regards to the patient disposition there is an argument this patient could be reviewed in either resuscitation room or majors, but resuscitation room would be most appropriate to allow for close observation and initiation of IV antihypertensive agents with continuous blood pressure monitoring.

☑ 2e Dilated ascending aorta, aortic arch and proximal descending aorta with filling defect suggestive of dissection

The mistake in this case would be to focus on the intracranial portion of the scan due to the patient history when in fact the most obvious and significant abnormality is a dissecting aneurysm of the ascending aorta, aortic arch and proximal descending aorta measuring 8 cm at its largest. The fact the patient is asymptomatic from an aortic aneurysm viewpoint suggests this may be a chronic pathology secondary to uncontrolled hypertension. The scan does also show a degree of small vessel disease but no evidence of acute intracranial infarct, which would be suggested by hypoattenuation and swelling. MRI would be the preferred imaging modality to assess further if there was a high suspicion of ischaemic stroke. Subarachnoid bleeding would be suggested by hyperdensity in the basal cisterns and fissures due to blood in the subarachnoid space, which may fill or partially fill sulci, fissures, cisterns and ventricles; sometimes this is seen layered over the tentorium, which causes it to appear denser than normal. The vertebral arteries are patent with no filling defects.

☑ 3c Group & screen, ensure two large bore cannulae, labetalol 2 mg per minute IV, refer to cardiothoracic team and intensive care unit (ICU)

The discovery of an aortic dissection with profound hypertension fits the criteria for a hypertensive emergency. This situation requires urgent IV antihypertensives with IV labetalol generally first line; it may be given as a bolus of 50 mg over 1 minute followed by a further 50 mg every 5 minutes until a satisfactory response occurs, or by continuous IV infusion. Infusion would allow for more controlled titration of blood pressure. The general treatment target in hypertensive emergencies is to produce a gradual, but prompt, reduction in blood pressure by 20–25% in the first 60 minutes with a target of ~160/100 mmHg. This is because lowering the BP too rapidly and/or by a significant amount in a patient with longstanding hypertension could result in organ hypoperfusion. However, in aortic dissection there is usually a more stringent blood pressure target of 120 mmHg systolic within 30 minutes. Patients requiring IV blood pressure control should be monitored in resuscitation room ideally with invasive blood pressure monitoring via an arterial line. Due to involvement of the proximal aorta, this is classified as a Stanford Type A dissection. Local guidelines may vary, but in general cardiothoracic surgeons manage Type A dissection as this may include involvement of the aortic root and valve, whereas vascular surgeons manage Type B. Patients who are fit enough would be considered for emergency surgery and those who are not would receive conservative medical management with stringent hypertensive control only.

KEY LEARNING POINTS

- CT head intracranial angiogram scans include an angiogram from the aortic arch, through the neck, into the cerebral arteries. Care should be taken to look for possible dissection as well as thrombus and atherosclerosis.
- Aggressive hypertension control is most easily achieved via IV agents such as labetalol with arterial line monitoring in a highly monitored environment.
- Proximal aortic dissections (ascending and arch) are usually managed by cardiothoracic surgeons surgically.

Sporting injury under the influence

A 26-year-old man is brought into the emergency department (ED) due to concerns of a hip fracture late in the evening. He tells you that he was running in a basketball court and landed awkwardly on his left foot. As he did so, he felt a sharp pain in his left hip and collapsed unable to get up. He tells you he had alcohol, cannabis and cocaine at approximately 1900 hours. Past medical history includes depression and a previous traumatic chest and bowel injury from a stabbing.

On examination the patient is in severe pain and appears to be under the mild influence of alcohol.

You perform a primary survey:

1. Airway and cervical spine: self-ventilating and no cervical spine pain
2. Breathing: RR 24, SpO_2 99% on room air, good air entry throughout both lungs
3. Circulation: HR 90, BP 125/75, abdomen soft, laparotomy scar noted, hips held in flexion with rolled blankets underneath
4. Disability: GCS 15/15, PEARLA 5 mm/5 mm, blood glucose 5.0 mmol/L
5. Exposure: there is no sign of external haemorrhage, both feet are warm and well perfused

The following radiographs were performed prior to your arrival, due to the suspicion of a hip fracture.

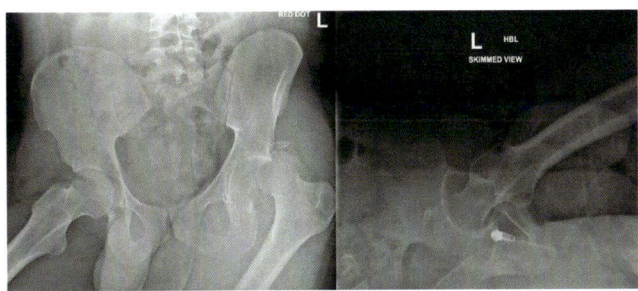

DOI: 10.1201/9781003461456-58

1. Which of the following best describes what is shown in the radiographs?

   a. Anterior dislocation of the left hip with an acetabular rim fracture

   b. Left acetabular blowout fracture

   c. Posterior dislocation of the left hip with an acetabular rim fracture

   d. Vertical shear injury to the left hip with disruption of the left SI joint

   e. Open book fracture with diastasis of the symphysis pubis

The patient is moved to the resuscitation room and a trauma call is activated. The primary survey is repeated and there are no new findings on examination.

Your team comprises of two anaesthetists, an orthopaedic registrar, a general surgical resident and two ED nurses. Ultrasound scanning is available.

The patient has now had 17.5 mg IV morphine and is still in 8/10 pain. The foot is still neurovascularly intact.

2. How would you proceed to deal with this injury?

   a. Ask the anaesthetic team to perform a femoral nerve block for pain relief and admit locally

   b. Perform a supra-inguinal fascia-iliaca block for pain relief and admit locally

   c. Give ketamine for pain relief and apply skin traction to the affected leg

   d. Apply a pelvic binder and transfer to the local major trauma centre

   e. Ask the anaesthetic team to sedate the patient and assist the orthopaedic registrar to reduce the injury

You remember a talk on hip fractures dividing the hip into two structural columns: the anterior and posterior column.

The orthopaedic surgeon highlighted a number of anatomical lines on a plain pelvic radiograph, which, when disrupted, could give you an indication of which column was injured.

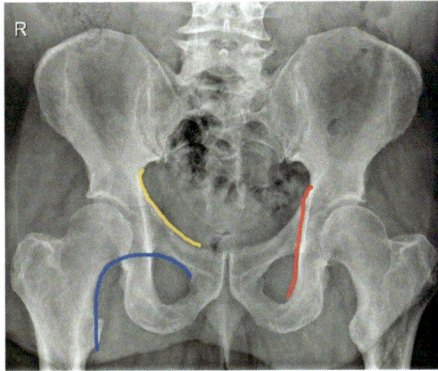

Yellow line: iliopectineal line; red: ilioshial line; blue: Shenton's line

3. Which of the following is the appropriately matched anatomical line and fracture pattern?

a. Iliopectineal line disruption: anterior column fracture

b. Ilioischial line disruption: acetabular fracture

c. Shenton's line disruption: acetabular fracture

d. Iliopectinal line disruption: posterior column fracture

e. Ilioischial line disruption: anterior column fracture

☑ 1c Posterior dislocation of the left hip with an acetabular rim fracture

The correct answer here is a posterior dislocation of the hip with an acetabular rim fracture. Posterior dislocations of the native hip are nine times more common than anterior dislocations of the hip. Normally, they are associated with high kinetic energy injuries such as passengers/drivers in a car whereby force is applied in an anteroposterior plane to a flexed hip. There is often an associated acetabular fracture as is the case here. The second most common injury mechanism is a sporting injury. Diagnosis is often clinical with key elements being a young patient, a compatible mechanism of injury and a characteristic flexion of the hip with extreme pain. Plain radiograph is sufficient to make the initial diagnosis with the lateral image helping to establish the direction of the femoral head. In patients where other injury is suspected, a CT polytrauma scan should be performed. Even in relatively straightforward cases, a CT pelvis will help to delineate the acetabular injury.

☑ 2e Ask the anaesthetic team to sedate the patient and assist the orthopaedic registrar to reduce the injury

The correct answer is the reduce the fracture with sedation as this will reduce the pressure on the surrounding neurovascular structures; remember the proximity of the sciatic nerve to the posterior gluteal region. You have a skilled team present with the right people to perform the procedure. Reduction is best achieved under deep sedation, for example with fentanyl and propofol, with full monitoring: ECG, SpO_2, non-invasive BP and waveform capnography. The most common reduction method is to apply traction anteriorly with the hip flexed, and with internal rotation. You may encounter resistance if the acetabular rim fracture is large and causes a mechanical block. Sometimes this procedure is best done in theatre under image intensifier (II) guidance and with the option to open the hip. Fascia-iliaca or femoral nerve block will only provide partial pain relief as the sciatic nerve is not blocked and may mask impending compartment syndrome. A pelvic binder is not indicated as this is not an open book fracture, and provided there are no other significant traumatic injuries, transferring to the major trauma centre is not indicated immediately.

☑ 3a Iliopectineal line disruption: anterior column fracture

The correct pairing is iliopectineal line: anterior column. The ilioischial line is associated with the posterior column. Shenton's line is not correct but is useful for looking for neck of femur fractures. The acetabulum is divided into two theoretical structural columns when looked at from laterally. These are the anterior column (anterior ilium, anterior wall and dome of the acetabulum, and superior pubic ramus) and the posterior column (greater and lesser sciatic notches, posterior wall and dome of the acetabulum and ischial tuberosity). Delineation of a serious column disruption is important to determine management of these fractures. CT is the best imaging modality to define this, but plain radiographs can give an initial impression. The iliopectineal line correlates with the pelvic brim for the anterior three-quarters and to the dense bone of the internal surface of the sciatic buttress (1–2 cm below the pelvic brim) for the posterior quarter. The ilioischial line is the result of the radiograph beam occurring in tangent across a segment of the surface of the quadrilateral plate.

KEY LEARNING POINTS

- Intoxication and substances that can alter judgement or coordination will often lead to more severe injuries even in young patients.
- Plain radiographs are usually sufficient to make the initial diagnosis of hip dislocation, but CT will provide additional detail such as concurrent acetabular injury.
- Reduction of native hip dislocations can be performed in the ED but will need safe deep sedation levels due to the need to overcome powerful hip and thigh muscles to allow successful manipulation.

CASE 59

Stridor

You are alerted by the ambulance service that they are transporting a patient to the emergency department as an inter-hospital transfer. They inform you he is a 55-year-old man with a background of squamous cell carcinoma of the soft palate. He has threatened airway obstruction, and they describe him as stridulous.

1. If stridor is present at rest, what is the estimated percentage of airway obstruction?
    a. 20%
    b. 40%
    c. 50%
    d. 80%
    e. 90%

On arrival, the patient is not compromised and you hear no stridor. You perform a primary survey after the paramedic handover.

Initial observations are recorded as HR 95, BP 138/98, SpO_2 95% on 1 L via nasal cannula, RR 28, temperature 36.8°C (98.2°F). On examination, the patient appears to be cushingoid, has a mildly increased work of breathing with accessory muscle use.

The documentation that arrives with the patient reads that he had a chest radiograph that was 'abnormal' but no further information is available.

A repeat portable chest radiograph is performed in the department.

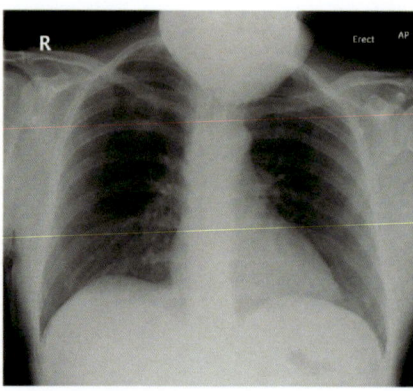

DOI: 10.1201/9781003461456-59

2. Which of the following would NOT be included in your differentials?

  a. Malignancy

  b. Staphylococcal pneumonia

  c. Rheumatoid arthritis

  d. Aspergilloma

  e. Silicosis

3. Considering the history and investigation results, which of the following would be the single best investigation to assist with a definitive diagnosis and plan for treatment in view of the chest radiograph findings?

  a. Nasendoscopy

  b. CT neck and CT chest with contrast

  c. CT neck and CT chest, abdomen & pelvis with contrast

  d. CT chest, abdomen & pelvis with contrast

  e. Bronchoscopy

☑ 1c 50%

Airway obstruction covers a spectrum of presentations and consists of upper airway obstruction (nose/mouth to larynx) and lower airway obstruction (tracheobronchial tree). Obstruction may be acute with severe signs and symptoms or more chronic where patients may have few symptoms until a sudden deterioration and 'tipping point'. Finally, obstruction may be complete or incomplete; complete obstruction of the upper airway is present if there is inability to talk, cough or breath. Incomplete obstruction occurs when there is partial upper airway obstruction and ability to breath is maintained. Inspiratory stridor and increased work of breathing are the hallmarks. Inspiratory stridor at rest implies reduction in airway diameter of approximately 50%. It is a serious sign and, in this patient, if present, could imply high risk of impending complete airway obstruction secondary to the oropharyngeal tumour. Management varies significantly based on the condition of the patient. Acute management in an awake patient with an element of inspiratory stridor can include high-flow nasal oxygen, steroid therapy (for example, dexamethasone 8 mg IV), nebulised adrenaline, Heliox (helium oxygen mixture) or CPAP as temporising measures.

☑ 2e Silicosis

The chest radiograph shows a thick-walled round cavity in the right upper lobe. The differential diagnoses of a cavitating lung lesion are wide, but pneumoconioses such as silicosis tend to cause calcified lesions rather than cavitating. In a patient with a known primary cancer, malignancy would be the primary differential (primary bronchogenic carcinoma, metastatic disease or local invasion could be considered in this patient's case). Other causes of pulmonary cavities include infection (pulmonary TB, cavitating pneumonia, which can be caused by *Staphylococcus aureus*, septic pulmonary emboli), non-infective granuloma (rheumatoid nodules, granulomatosis with polyangiitis), pulmonary infarction or traumatic pneumatocoele.

☑ 3c CT neck and CT chest, abdomen & pelvis with contrast

Cross-sectional imaging is required to assess the primary oropharyngeal cancer (CT neck) and assess the lesion noted on the chest radiograph (CT chest). Additionally, CT abdomen & pelvis should be performed for staging to assess for any additional distant metastatic disease. Bronchoscopy could be considered later in the investigation of suspected lung mass after cross-sectional imaging to obtain a biopsy. Note that performing bronchoscopy could prove challenging, however, in a patient with head and neck cancer, due to anatomical changes secondary to the tumour and previous treatment (for example, scarring following radiotherapy). Nasendoscopy is quick and easily performed at the bedside by the ENT or head and neck surgery team and can provide a lot of information about the appearance of the airway. However, it will not provide information regarding spread of the cancer, nor any information regarding the lung lesion. Therefore, if the patient is stable enough to transfer to CT and can lie flat, this will provide greater information and allow a treatment plan to be instigated by the parent team.

KEY LEARNING POINTS

- Stridor at rest implies airflow obstruction of at least 50% and should be taken seriously.
- The differentials for a cavitating lung lesion are wide and include malignancy, bacterial infections, fungal infections and rheumatological disorders such as rheumatoid arthritis.
- Both radiological assessment of cancer spread and a tissue diagnosis are essential components for planning definitive treatment. When performing axial imaging in the ED, consider the need to widen scan parameters for subsequent treatment.

CASE 60

Swollen eye

A 5-year-old girl presents to the emergency department (ED) with her mother, complaining of unilateral eye swelling. Her mother informs you that since waking this morning she has been itching her right eye, and a few hours later she noticed redness and a thin discharge in the corners of it. She is otherwise well in herself, has no other symptoms and has not been febrile. She has no significant past medical history, and immunisations are up to date. There have been no previous safeguarding concerns or contact with social services.

Initial observations are recorded as HR 102, SpO_2 97% on room air, RR 29, temperature 37.7°C (99.8°F).

On examination, the patient looks generally well and is active, playing with her sister. There is evident swelling and erythema of the right upper and lower eyelid, and she can just about open her eye passively – see clinical photo.

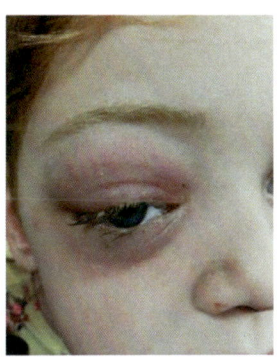

The globe itself appears normal, there is no obvious visual impairment and no pain on eye movements. There is no proptosis. The remainder of systemic examinations are normal.

DOI: 10.1201/9781003461456-60

Bloods are taken and you review the results.

White cell count	23.23^
Red cell count	4.39
Haemoglobin	125
HCT	0.346ᵥ
MCV	78.8
MCH	28.5
MCHC (g/L)	361^
RDW	11.9
Platelet count	516^
MPV	9.7
Neutrophils	19.54^
Lymphocytes	1.42ᵥ
Monocytes	2.21^
Eosinophils	0.00ᵥ
Basophils	0.07
XE Nucleated…	0.00
XE Nucleated…	0.0
C-reactive protein	150.3^

1. Based on the clinical examination findings and initial investigation results, which of the following is the most likely diagnosis?

   a. Non-accidental injury

   b. Allergic rhinitis

   c. Orbital cellulitis

   d. Periorbital cellulitis

   e. Nephrotic syndrome

The patient is reviewed by the ophthalmology team in the ED, given a dose of IV ceftriaxone and discharged to continue outpatient IV antibiotics with clear advice on when to return.

Her mother brings her back to the ED the following morning as overnight the child experienced high fevers with worsening of the eye swelling. She is now unable to open her right eye and is complaining of pain around the area. Her mother reports that she is not herself and has not been wanting to eat this morning.

An urgent CT orbits with contrast is arranged.

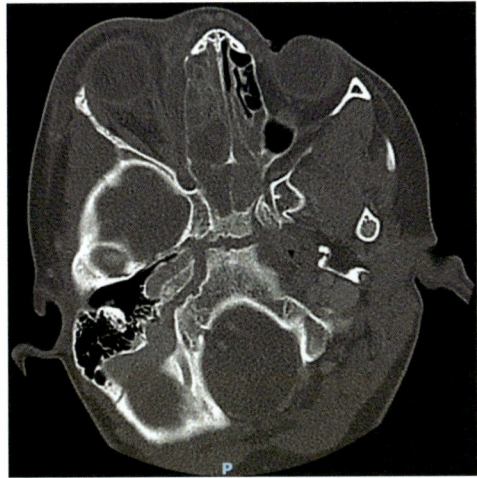

2. Which of the following is the best description of the findings seen on this CT?

   a. Appearances appear suspicious of an optic nerve glioma

   b. There is an enhancing collection along the right medial extraconal orbit with an intracranial extension to a large collection in the right anterior cranial fossa around a locule of pneumocephalus

   c. There is an enhancing collection along the right medial extraconal orbit; appearances are suspicious for a subperiosteal abscess

   d. There is enhancing collection along both the right and left medial extraconal orbit

   e. There is no opacification of the right maxillary, ethmoidal and sphenoid chambers

You review the literature surrounding the role of endoscopic endonasal surgery in the operative management of anterior skull base pathology.

3. Which of the following is the most common complication associated with this procedure?

   a. CSF leak

   b. Astrocytoma

   c. Intracranial infection

   d. Cranial nerve VI palsy

   e. Cranial nerve III palsy

☑ 1d Periorbital cellulitis

The clinical examination findings of periorbital swelling and erythema, along with the evidence of raised inflammatory markers, point to a diagnosis of periorbital cellulitis. The presence of pain on eye movement, deep ocular pain and proptosis (which can be subtle), would suggest a true orbital cellulitis; this is an important differential to exclude at this stage. Patients with orbital cellulitis often appear systemically unwell with high fevers, and may display diplopia, ophthalmoplegia, chemosis and visual impairment. However, given that orbital cellulitis is sight-threatening and that it can be difficult to differentiate the two, always err on the side of caution. Allergic rhinitis may present with pruritus and erythema, but generally would not cause significant unilateral swelling. In nephrotic syndrome there is typically bilateral generalised facial oedema without erythema. Neither allergic rhinitis or nephrotic syndrome would explain the raised inflammatory markers. Additionally, to confirm nephrotic syndrome you would need urinalysis and albumin levels. Non-accidental injury is something to always have in the back of your mind, but there do not appear to be any red flags in the history to make this diagnosis more likely, and again this would not necessarily lead to deranged blood results.

☑ 2c There is an enhancing collection along the right medial extraconal orbit; appearances are suspicious for a subperiosteal abscess

The abnormality in this CT orbits is quite subtle, but there is a collection along the right medial extraconal orbital region. This is highly suspicious of a subperiosteal abscess. Additionally, the right maxillary and ethmoidal, and both sphenoid sinuses, are opacified. These features are very typical of orbital cellulitis. Furthermore, there is a small enhancing focus within the floor of the anterior cranial fossa, which may represent intracranial extension. However, there is no large collection within the anterior cranial fossa, and no evidence of pneumocephalus. The left medial extraconal orbit appears normal. An optic nerve glioma would be suggested by enlargement of the optic nerve and canal; the optic nerve may also be seen as kinked or buckled. If these features were present, an MRI should be arranged to assess further.

☑ 3a CSF leak

The most commonly reported complication associated with endoscopic endonasal surgery is CSF leak, which can cause symptoms of low-pressure headache, neck pain and stiffness, photophobia, tinnitus and ringing in the ear and occasionally loss of smell or taste. CSF leak also increases risk of meningitis, pneumocephalus, acute subdural haemorrhage and cerebellar sag. Risk factors for CSF leak include pre-operative hydrocephalus, obesity, operative site and surgeon experience. Other complications of endoscopic endonasal surgery include bleeding and haematoma, intracranial infection (including meningitis), internal carotid artery injury, pituitary gland dysfunction and cranial nerve dysfunction. Isolated abducens nerve palsy is the most common cranial nerve pathology due to its location and trajectory. Neuromonitoring during the procedure can be cost effective and help to identify cranial nerves during surgery, but there are benefits and limitations to each modality.

KEY LEARNING POINTS

- Differentiating between periorbital cellulitis and orbital cellulitis can be difficult. It is always best to seek expert opinion to avoid potential sight- and brain-threatening infection.
- CT orbits is a readily available and quick imaging modality to assess for orbital cellulitis and despite the radiation risk this is preferred over MRI due to availability and less need for sedation.
- CSF leak can commonly occur with endoscopic endonasal anterior skull base surgery, which itself can increase risk of further complications.

Swollen knees

A 38-year-old man is brought to the emergency department by ambulance after falling from an e-scooter. He was travelling at around 20 mph but confused the brake with accelerator and came to a sudden halt, falling forwards and landing with knees first onto the ground. He denies head injury or any other injuries but reports significant pain in both knees after feeling 'explosions' and is unable to straight leg raise either leg from the bed. He is unable to weight-bear in the department. Past medical history includes end-stage renal failure on haemodialysis 3 times per week.

Bilateral knee radiographs are performed.

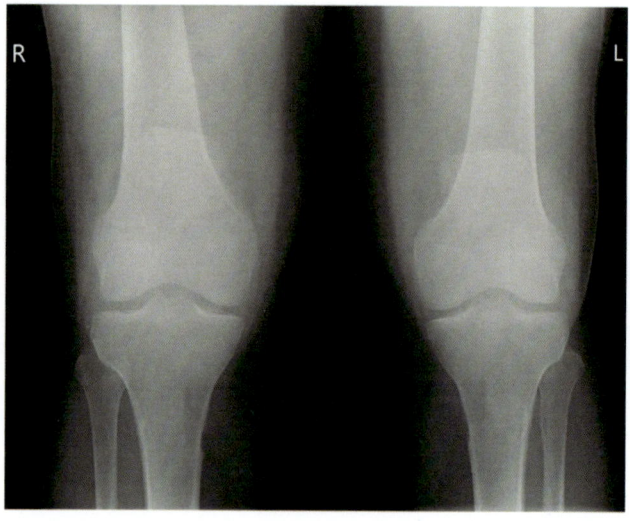

1. Which of the following is the best interpretation of the radiographs?
   a. Bilateral patella tendon rupture
   b. Right patella fracture
   c. Left medial tibia plateau fracture
   d. Normal radiograph
   e. Bilateral quadriceps tendon rupture

DOI: 10.1201/9781003461456-61

2. Which of the following is a potential precipitating factor to his injuries?

    a. Immunosuppressants

    b. Osteomalacia

    c. Osteoarthritis of the knee

    d. Steroid use and renal failure

    e. Osgood–Schlatter disease

3. Which of the following is the best management plan for this patient?

    a. Advise 'rest, ice, compression and elevation' and refer to outpatient fracture clinic

    b. Reduction under sedation, cylinder cast and refer to outpatient fracture clinic

    c. Apply above knee backslab and refer to orthopaedics for surgical management

    d. Apply AirCast boots and refer to outpatient orthopaedics for review

    e. Refer to acute internal medicine team for admission, renal review and urgent MRI knees

☑ 1a Bilateral patella tendon rupture

This radiograph shows bilateral patella tendon rupture. The key, as always, is in the history here; if the patient cannot straight leg raise, then the extensor mechanism is disrupted – in other words, the quadriceps or its tendon, the patella itself or the patella tendon and or its insertion. Looking carefully at the images, both patellae appear to be superiorly translated. This is known as 'patella alta' or high patella as a direct translation from Latin. It is easy to miss and often patients are incorrectly sent to fracture clinic in a cricket pad splint and crutches. On the lateral view, the Insall–Salvati ratio can be measured to determine if the patella is high: patella tendon length divided by patella length with a normal value between 0.8 and 1.2. Values greater than 1.2 equate to patella alta. Remember that if the quadriceps tendon is ruptured, the patella may appear to be in a normal position, but the clue may be in a palpable defect just superior to the patella. There is no discontinuity of bone cortex, step or presence of abnormal fat pads on this AP radiograph, which could indicate fracture.

☑ 2d Steroid use and renal failure

Corticosteroid use has been linked to an increase in tendon weakness, whether given systemically or by local infiltration. This in combination with chronic renal failure, specifically uraemia, may have contributed to this patient's injury. Other risk factors include diabetes mellitus, systemic lupus erythematous and rheumatoid arthritis, which can all weaken collagen structure, patellar tendinopathy or degeneration or previous patella injury. The mechanism of injury is also important and is most commonly tensile overload of the extensor (sudden quadriceps contraction with knee flexed, for example jumping or missing a step on stairs). The greatest force on the tendon is when the knee if flexed to >60 degrees. Considering the other answer options, osteomalacia is caused by vitamin D or calcium deficiency, or genetic defect. It can present with bone pain, muscle weakness and risk of fractures. Osgood–Schlatter disease is due to inflammation below the knee where the patellar tendon inserts to the tibia. It is common in adolescents during growth spurts and often responds to conservative management whereby symptoms completely resolve without any complications over time and with reduced sporting activity.

☑ 3c Apply above knee backslab and refer to orthopaedics for surgical management

Patella tendon rupture management depends on whether this is partial or complete. Partial tendon rupture is usually treated non-operatively with knee brace and non-weight-bearing crutches initially, followed by graded weight-bearing as tolerated for 3–6 weeks. Complete tendon rupture is usually treated with operative repair, non-weight-bearing with knee brace and crutches post-operatively. The particular indication for surgical management in this case is the presence of bilateral rupture. Shorter time to surgical repair is associated with better outcomes of recovery and lower incidence of quadriceps weakness and incomplete knee flexion post-operatively. Almost all cases of patella tendon rupture require orthopaedic input, but in particular if there are any of the following: associated fracture (for example, tibial plateau, patella); paediatric patients (sleeve fractures are often missed due to cartilaginous tendon attachment in children); or expected non-compliance with knee immobilisation or non-weight-bearing status. MRI or ultrasound may be indicated if differentiation between partial and complete rupture is required; the need for this should be guided by the orthopaedic team.

KEY LEARNING POINTS

- Patella tendon rupture is easy to miss radiologically but clinical inability to straight-leg raise should prompt formal measurement of the Insall–Salvati ratio on the radiograph.
- Chronic steroid use and renal failure are significant risk factors for tendon weakening.
- Surgical management should be considered for bilateral patella tendon ruptures and those who have a high risk anaesthetic profile.

CASE 62

Symptomatic hypotension

A 59-year-old woman presents to the emergency department after seeing her GP due to light-headedness. At the GP surgery she was noted to be hypotensive on standing and an ambulance was arranged. She describes dizziness starting after lifting something heavy off the floor the previous day, which is associated with dyspnoea and mid-scapular pain that radiates to the left anterior chest. She denies cough, coryza or fever.

Initial observations are recorded as HR 78, BP 109/55, SpO_2 97% on room air, RR 21, temperature 36.8°C (98.2°F). Cardiac, respiratory and abdominal examinations do not reveal any abnormalities.

A venous blood gas (VBG) is performed and reveals pH 7.416, pCO_2 5.44, HCO_3^- 23.8, BE +1.7, Lactate 2.7, Hb 140.

The initial ECG is shown.

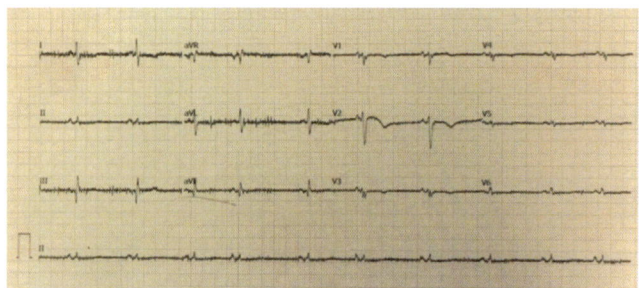

1. Which of the following diagnoses is best suggested by this ECG?
    a. Posterior myocardial infarction
    b. Pacemaker dysfunction
    c. Normal ECG
    d. Massive pulmonary embolus
    e. Wellens' syndrome

On review of the laboratory blood results, you note Hb 133, WCC 9.06, Troponin T 57, D-dimer 2480, normal renal function.

DOI: 10.1201/9781003461456-62

She now complains of worsening pain between the scapulae, and blood pressure has fallen to 89/59.

A CT aortogram is performed.

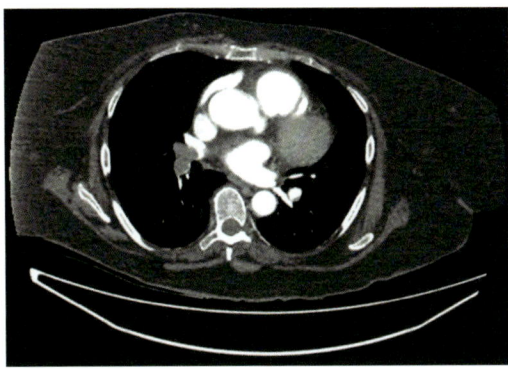 

2. Based on the provided investigation results, which of the following is the best management option?

   a. Administer treatment dose low molecular weight heparin, discharge to be reviewed in the acute internal medicine hot clinic

   b. Move to the resuscitation room for thrombolysis with alteplase 50 mg IV stat

   c. Administer aspirin 300 mg PO, clopidogrel 300 mg PO, fondaparinux 2.5 mg SC and refer to acute internal medicine

   d. Arrange time-critical transfer to cardiothoracic surgeons for urgent surgical intervention

   e. Move to the resuscitation room for thrombolysis with alteplase 1.5 mg/kg (max 100 mg) – 10 mg IV stat & remainder over 2 hours

Following the CT, the patient's blood pressure remains low with systolic BP ranging between 80 and 90 mmHg.

3. Which of the following statements is correct?

   a. Give repeated 500 mL colloid boluses only to manage hypotension

   b. Thrombolytic therapy does not reduce residual dyspnoea or RV dysfunction in the long term

   c. Catheter-directed thrombolysis can be performed when systemic thrombolysis is absolutely contraindicated

   d. Surgical embolectomy should not be considered

   e. In the case of cardiac arrest, CPR should be discontinued after 10 minutes

☑ 1d Massive pulmonary embolus

The above ECG is tricky to interpret due to the poor baseline caused by artefact. However, there is a prominent S wave in lead I and deep Q waves in III. There are T waves present in lead III alternating between flat and normal morphology. The overall suggestion is that of acute pulmonary embolus based on the ECG and clinical findings. Right-sided precordial and inferior lead T-wave inversion is indicative of a right ventricular strain pattern associated with high pulmonary pressures, seen in ~35% of patients with PE. These two findings together should direct you to massive PE as a likely diagnosis. Posterior MI accompanies 15–20% of STEMI (usually in the context of lateral or inferior infarction); isolated posterior MI is less common (3–11%). The typical pattern of ST elevation is inverted leading to the following changes in V1–3: ST elevation becomes ST depression, Q waves become R waves, terminal T-wave inversion becomes an upright T wave. A useful tip is to turn the ECG over and upside-down and hold it up to the light. Wellens' syndrome is a pattern of deeply inverted or biphasic T waves in V2–3, which is highly specific for a critical stenosis of the left anterior descending artery (LAD). The ECG of aortic dissection can be normal, be associated with ST elevation inferiorly if the right coronary artery is involved, be suggestive of pericarditis, or display electrical alternans (if tamponade present).

☑ 2e Move to the resuscitation room for thrombolysis with alteplase 1.5 mg/kg (max 100 mg) – 10 mg IV stat & remainder over 2 hours

This CT shows extensive bilateral PEs within the distal parts of both main pulmonary arteries extending to lobar, segmental and subsegmental pulmonary artery branches. The burden of emboli in this patient is severe with involvement of all lobes. There is inverse interventricular septal deviation indicating significant right heart strain. The aorta appears normal and there is no dissection. The sPESI (Simplified Pulmonary Embolism Severity Index) score can be used to help predict 30-day outcome of patients with PE. It has fewer criteria than the original PESI score: a score of 1 or greater predicts higher severity (up to 8.9% mortality). Due to the hypotension and extensive emboli with right ventricular strain this patient is high risk and therefore thrombolysis is first line treatment. Alteplase is a fibrin-specific tissue plasminogen activator. The dose for alteplase in the British National Formulary (BNF) is 10 mg over 1–2 minutes, followed by an infusion of 90 mg over 2 hours, with a maximum dose of 1.5 mg/kg in patients less than 65 kg. However, there is some evidence to suggest that 50 mg alteplase has identical efficacy compared to 100 mg, with fewer bleeding complications. At present, more research is needed in this area, but the current best practice is the dosing described above.

☑ 3b Thrombolytic therapy does not reduce residual dyspnoea or RV dysfunction in the long term

Studies have shown approximately one third of patients report some persistent functional limitation, and that thrombolytic treatment did not improve long-term mortality rates or reduce residual RV dysfunction or symptoms of dyspnoea. Contraindications to catheter-directed thrombolysis are the same as those for systemic thrombolysis and include active bleeding or known bleeding disorder, recent intracranial or spinal surgery, recent trauma, history of haemorrhagic stroke or non-haemorrhagic stroke in the previous 3 months. However, catheter-directed thrombolysis can be performed when there is a relative contraindication to systemic thrombolysis, which includes severe uncontrolled hypertension, non-haemorrhagic stroke more than 3 months prior, pregnancy and surgery within the last 10–14 days. Catheter-directed thrombectomy can be performed in patients with absolute contraindications to thrombolytics or failed thrombolytic therapy, with open-surgical embolectomy reserved for high-risk patients with absolute contraindications or failed thrombolytic therapy, cardiogenic shock with risk of death prior to thrombolytic therapy, or thrombus in right heart or across patent foramen ovale. There is risk that thrombolytic therapy could fail and therefore catheter-directed or surgical embolectomy would be considered for this patient. In the presence of shock, fluid resuscitation is not recommended unless there is definitive evidence of co-existing hypovolaemia; vasopressors should be used to stabilise BP until thrombolysis. In cardiac arrest due to PE or where there is high suspicion of PE, give alteplase 50 mg IV bolus and continue CPR for at least 60 minutes.

KEY LEARNING POINTS

- There are a myriad of ECG signs that suggest an acute pulmonary embolus, ranging from sinus tachycardia to right-heart strain patterns (right axis deviation, S-waves in V5/6 and III).
- Systemic thrombolysis should be considered for massive pulmonary embolus or patients displaying haemodynamic instability in the absence of contraindications.
- A range of other treatment options now exist for treating pulmonary emboli, and multidisciplinary team input from acute internal medicine physicians, haematology, interventional radiology and cardiothoracic surgeons can help in complex cases.

CASE 63

Testicular pain

A 33-year-old man presents to the emergency department. He complains of scrotal pain and swelling for the last 3 days. He tells you that he is normally fit and well but has a past medical history of hidradenitis suppurativa. He works in the hospitality industry and can spend significant periods of time sitting.

Initial observations are recorded as HR 105, BP 161/105, SpO$_2$ 98% on room air, RR 19, temperature 36.6°C (97.9°F), CBG 15.7. The patient appears to be sweating profusely. You note a raised body mass index. Examination of the external genitalia and perineum with a chaperone present reveals a hardened indurated mass to the right scrotum. The testes are palpable, but assessment is limited due to significant pain. Cremasteric reflex is tricky to elicit.

Point-of-care urine dipstick on midstream urine (MSU) sample shows glucose 4+ and trace ketones and is sent for microscopy and culture.

1. Which of the following are the best next immediate steps with this patient?
   a. Discharge with oral flucloxacillin 500 mg QDS 7 days
   b. Discharge with clindamycin 600 mg QDS 7 days
   c. FBC/U&E/CRP/VBG, refer to urology and add on a HbA1c
   d. FBC/U&E/CRP/VBG, start variable rate insulin infusion, refer to urology
   e. FBC/U&E/CRP/coagulation/VBG, refer to urology for immediate de-torsion

An urgent ultrasound scrotum is arranged for the patient, and he returns for review.

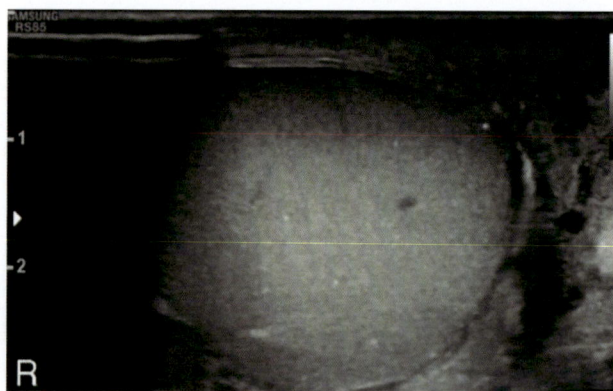

DOI: 10.1201/9781003461456-63

2. What does the imaging suggest?

   a. Microlithiasis

   b. Varicocele

   c. Acute torsion with small reactive hydrocoele

   d. Scrotal abscess

   e. Fournier's gangrene with gas forming organisms

3. Which of the following conditions may be associated with the above sonographic findings?

   a. Trauma

   b. Varicocele

   c. Sexually transmitted infections

   d. Germ cell carcinoma of the testis

   e. Diabetes mellitus

☑   1c FBC/U&E/CRP/VBG, refer to urology and add on a HbA1c

There are two elements to the clinical history. Firstly, the patient has a high body mass index, and you note that the blood sugar is elevated at 15.7 mmol/L with glycosuria and trace ketonuria. This would be in keeping with undiagnosed type 2 diabetes mellitus. A venous blood gas (VBG) would further clarify his metabolic state and in the absence of significant metabolic acidosis the key treatment would be to start metformin 500 mg once daily after measuring his eGFR. Remember a sliding scale is typically indicated in type 1 diabetics who are being fasted, for example before surgery, and not yet in this case. Secondly, the patient has a history of hidradenitis suppurativa, which is strongly linked to obesity and smoking, hence predisposing this patient to deep and painful abscesses. The worry here is that although the observations are 'relatively' normal, the patient looks clinically unwell, and this may signify deep infection.

☑   2a Microlithiasis

As the radiologist sweeps across the right testicle, you can see the pampiniform plexus in the first few seconds of the video and then the body of the testis. The striking abnormalities are the numerous tiny microcalcifications that appear to twinkle like stars. This is microlithiasis, a rare and often asymptomatic finding in about 1–5% of healthy men. In contrast, a varicocele would appear as a mass of engorged veins and a scrotal abscess as an organised hypoechoic collection. The presence of gas in the tissues, presenting as multiple hypoechoic dots, should immediately raise concern for Fournier's gangrene, which is a surgical emergency. Testicular torsion is a urological emergency caused by twisting of the testis on the spermatic cord, which constricts the vascular supply and can lead to ischaemia and/or necrosis of the tissue. It is most often a clinical diagnosis, and if history and examination suggest torsion, immediate surgical exploration should be arranged. Adding colour Doppler can help in aiding the diagnosis of torsion (no signal suggests torsion). There may be other non-specific features such as swelling, reduced echogenicity and a reactive hydrocele.

☑   3d Germ cell carcinoma of the testis

Microlithiasis is a rare condition that is mostly benign. It is commonly found on routine ultrasound of the testis and is usually bilateral. The appearances can range from a few uniformly scattered stones to very heavy loads that can give a 'snowstorm' appearance on ultrasound. They are thought to be a marker of tubular degeneration. It is present in around 50% of men with a germ cell tumour of the testis. Yearly routine follow-up is recommended for men with additional risks for germ cell carcinoma such as maldescent, orchidopexy, testicular atrophy, personal or family history of germ cell carcinoma. Other associations of microlithiasis include subfertility, Klinefelter syndrome and Down syndrome.

KEY LEARNING POINTS

- When the diagnosis of testicular torsion or abscess is unclear clinically, ultrasound can help clarify the diagnosis.
- Microlithiasis is often an incidental finding on testicular ultrasound and is thought to be a marker of tubular degeneration.
- Very rarely, microlithiasis is associated with germ cell tumours of the testis. Yearly follow-up surveillance scanning and self-examination are recommended.

CASE 64

They told me to do it

A 33-year-old man presents to the emergency department with burning epigastric pain radiating into the chest and states he has ingested something with the intention of harming himself. He has a history of schizophrenia, depression and self-harm. For the last couple of days, he states he has been hearing voices telling him to hurt himself.

Initial observations are recorded as HR 88, BP 123/61, SpO_2 98% on room air, RR 16, temperature 36.6°C (97.9°C). On examination, the abdomen is soft but tender in the epigastrium.

A venous blood gas (VBG) is performed which reveals pH 7.375, K^+ 3.7, Na^+ 143, Ca^{2+} 1.22, Cl^- 107, Glucose 5.1, lactate 0.9, BE 4.0, HCO_3^- 25.8.

The ECG shows sinus rhythm, QTc = 388 ms.

SADPERSONS score = 7

A chest radiograph is performed.

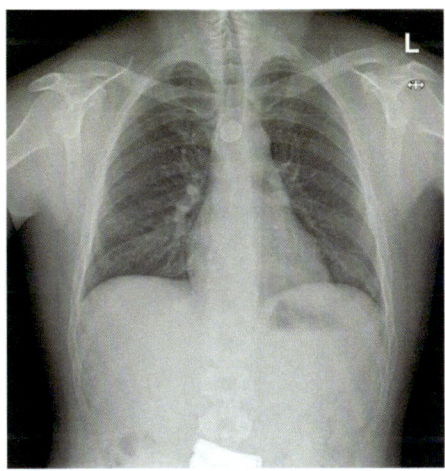

DOI: 10.1201/9781003461456-64

1. Based on the examination findings and chest radiograph, which of the following would be your next management step?

   a. Discharge to mental health with advice to attend acute internal medicine hot clinic for repeat radiograph in 72 hours

   b. Draw bloods, admit under the general surgery team for observation and/or proceed to laparotomy

   c. Draw bloods, admit under gastroenterology, give intravenous proton-pump inhibitor and prokinetic agent (for example, metoclopramide)

   d. Draw bloods, keep NBM, admit under gastroenterology for urgent OGD, refer to liaison mental health team for parallel assessment

   e. Draw bloods, keep NBM, admit under acute internal medicine for serial radiograph examinations, refer to liaison mental health team for next day review

The patient's pain worsens, and a CT chest, abdomen & pelvis is performed.

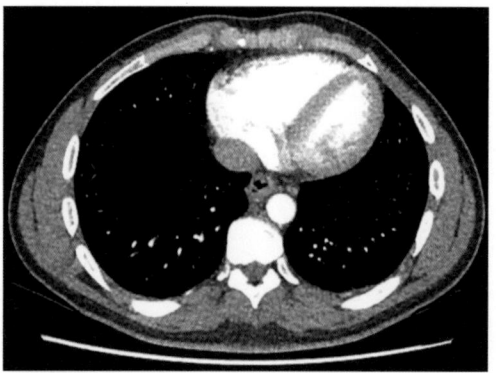

2. What is the best description of the findings shown on the CT?

   a. There is evidence of an oesophageal-aortal fistula with evidence of early contained leak; urgent cardiothoracic referral is advised

   b. There is evidence of oedema to the mid-oesophagus but no evidence of perforation; at least three foreign bodies now appear to lie within the gastric fundus

   c. There is evidence of passage of the foreign bodies visualised on the chest radiograph, which all now appear to lie within the proximal small bowel; follow-up with serial abdominal radiograph is recommended

   d. There is evidence of pancreatic inflammation and oedema suggestive of acute pancreatitis; gastroenterology opinion is advised as well as correlation with serum amylase levels

   e. There appears to be a well-rounded, metallic foreign body in the trachea just above the carina; urgent respiratory opinion and bronchoscopy is advised

The patient has a subsequent OGD as part of his inpatient stay.

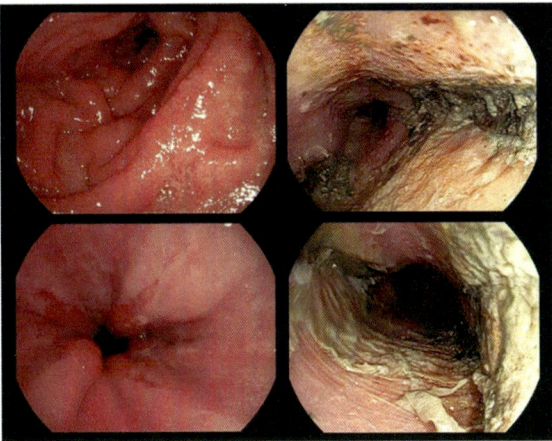 

3. Which type of foreign body is most likely to have caused the lesions shown?

   a. AA alkaline cell

   b. C zinc-carbon cell

   c. AA nickel metal hydride cell

   d. Lithium polymer cell

   e. Lithium or alkaline coin cell

☑ 1d Draw bloods, keep NBM, admit under gastroenterology for urgent OGD, refer to liaison mental health team for parallel assessment

This is an unusual case in an adult patient. There is a coin cell lodged in the oesophagus and two cylindrical cells (AA) in the stomach. Lateral chest radiograph, or better still, CT may be required if there is doubt whether the battery has been ingested (oesophagus) or aspirated (trachea). The lithium coin cell is the priority and should be treated as a medical emergency. Death can occur in as little as 2 hours post-ingestion. The initial assessment of the patient should include mental health risk stratification (for example, SADPERSONS score), capacity assessment and medical assessment. You should consider performing both chest and abdominal radiographs to image the number of objects potentially ingested and in this case, refer urgently to gastroenterology for OGD as the coin cell appears to be lodged in the oesophagus. Mental health assessment should occur in parallel to the medical care as Mental Health Act assessment (section) may be required for medical treatment in the case of acute psychosis.

☑ 2b There is evidence of oedema to the mid-oesophagus but no evidence of perforation; at least three foreign bodies now appear to lie within the gastric fundus

The main indication for performing this CT with contrast is the concern of perforation or fistulation. Following the images down, one can appreciate the trachea lying anteriorly in the mediastinum with the oesophagus immediately behind it. The coin cell seems to have passed through the oesophagus now but there is thickening in the mid-section indicating acute oedema secondary to the coin cell leaking (see around 12 seconds on the video clip). There is no contrast leak to indicate a fistula or any mediastinal free air. As the CT progresses into the upper abdomen, the batteries appear in one group lying in the fundus of the stomach (39 seconds on the video). The 'starburst' artefact is caused by the metal jacket of the AA cells, but they have not as yet passed into the duodenum or small bowel. There is no evidence of pancreatic inflammation in the portion imaged or any evidence of intra-abdominal free air.

☑ 3e Lithium or alkaline coin cell

The OGD images show severe corrosive injury to the oesophageal mucosa. Contact with the negative electrode causes a tiny current to pass and the formation of sodium hydroxide (alkali). Larger cells (>20 mm) are at increased risk of getting lodged within the oesophagus and complications include perforation and aortic fistulation. In asymptomatic patients, if the coin cell is beyond the oesophagus and <20 mm, patients can be considered for expectant management and discharge with clear advice for when to return and a follow-up plan in place. Coin cells lodged in the oesophagus or trachea should be removed immediately via endoscopy irrespective of symptoms. Cylindrical cells can cause problems if damaged prior to ingestion, for example by chewing. Whole, undamaged cylindrical cells can be managed expectantly with serial radiographs in asymptomatic patients if the battery has passed into the stomach at time of initial imaging; however, all cases should be referred to gastroenterology or general surgery for assessment. Be aware that perforation can still occur as a late complication after removal of all batteries and therefore patients and care givers must be given clear advice about when to return, and if they do come back, concerns should be taken seriously.

KEY LEARNING POINTS

- Have a low threshold for imaging patients who allege deliberate or unintentional ingestion of foreign bodies. Degree of radio-opaqueness, age and risk factors will determine the correct imaging modality.
- Refer early to mental health teams in parallel as the assessment and treatment of the acute psychosis is as important as the medical treatment. In addition, Mental Health Act sections may be required if the patient cannot consent to treatment.
- Coin cell ingestion is a medical emergency. Take all suspected ingestion seriously and image early due to the risk of corrosive injury and perforation.

Thigh pain

A 34-year-old man presents to the emergency department with painful right thigh swelling. This developed after he tried to inject heroin and a 'fat-burner' into a capillary 10 days ago. He has been taking oral flucloxacillin from his GP, but symptoms have worsened, and he is now unable to walk.

Initial observations are recorded as HR 104, BP 150/74, SpO$_2$ 96% on room air, RR 19, temperature 37.1°C (98.8°F). On examination, there is a 30 cm x 30 cm erythematous swelling on the right anterior thigh, which is warm to touch and tender to light palpation. Deep palpation demonstrates some fluctuance, but there is no surgical emphysema. There is a slightly reduced range of motion of the knee but no pain in the calf. Distal neurovascular examination is normal.

You mark the erythema on the skin and take a clinical photo after consent.

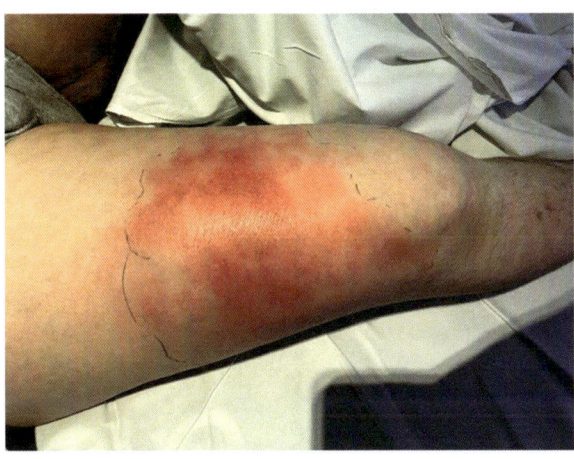

1. Which one clinical diagnosis is LEAST likely based on these findings?
   a. Cellulitis
   b. Below knee deep vein thrombosis (DVT)
   c. Intramuscular abscess
   d. Necrotising fasciitis
   e. Erysipelas

DOI: 10.1201/9781003461456-65

He is referred to the orthopaedic team who admit him and arrange an MRI scan of his right thigh.

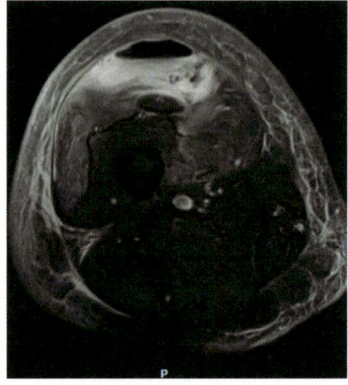

2. Which of the following best describes the findings that are present on these images?

  a. Fluid collection within medial compartment musculature with a gas-fluid level and breach of deep fascia

  b. Fluid collection within the anterior compartment musculature with synovial enhancement and thickening

  c. Fluid collection within the medial compartment musculature with a gas-fluid level and bone marrow oedema of the distal femur

  d. Fluid collection within the medial compartment musculature with synovial enhancement and thickening

  e. Fluid collection within anterior compartment musculature with a gas-fluid level and breach of superficial fascia

The patient is taken to theatre the next day and the following samples are collected.

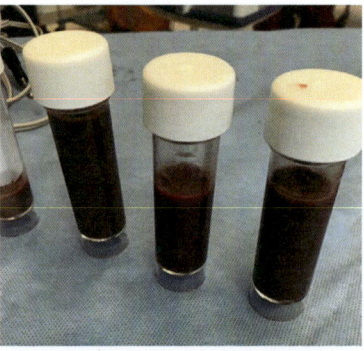

The fluid culture grows both Gram-positive cocci and Gram-negative bacilli at 24 hours. The patient has no reported drug allergy.

3. Which of the following empirical intravenous antibiotic regimens would provide the most appropriate cover prior to organism identification and sensitivities?

   a. Ciprofloxacin 400 mg BD + Clindamycin 600 mg QDS + Benzylpenicillin 1.2 g QDS

   b. Ciprofloxacin 400 mg BD + Clindamycin 600 mg QDS + Teicoplanin 400 mg OD

   c. Flucloxacillin 2 g QDS + Benzylpenicillin 1.2 g QDS

   d. Ciprofloxacin 400 mg BD + Clindamycin 600 mg QDS + Flucloxacillin 2 g QDS

   e. Ciprofloxacin 400 mg BD + Clindamycin 600 mg QDS

☑ 1b Below knee deep vein thrombosis

This patient has a large warm swelling of the anterior thigh affecting movement of the knee joint suggesting that there is involvement of the underlying musculature. This could be suggestive of intramuscular abscess. There are no classical features that provoke high suspicion of necrotising fasciitis, but it should always be considered. Features of necrotising fasciitis can include smooth shiny and tensely swollen skin; dark patches, blisters and bullae; crepitus; severe pain out of proportion to clinical findings; cutaneous anaesthesia; systemically unwell. The examination findings do not suggest any involvement of the knee joint itself, so a septic arthritis is a less likely cause, but the limited range of motion in this joint should make you consider this. Erysipelas is a bacterial infection of the skin caused by *Streptococcus pyogenes* and characteristically has a bright 'fire-like' appearance. Lastly, below knee (distal) DVT are isolated to the calf veins and so the photo of anterior thigh swelling makes this the least likely diagnosis.

☑ 2e Fluid collection within anterior compartment musculature with a gas-fluid level and breach of superficial fascia

This is a proton density sequence where fluid is seen as white, and air is seen as black. It is used by radiologists to assess potential joint involvement. Looking at the MRI, within the anterior compartment of the thigh, there is a large complex fluid collection breaching rectus femoris and vastus with a gas-fluid level and multiple gas locules. There is also an associated breach of the anterior superficial fascia, but this does not extend down into the knee joint and synovium. Remember that the thigh is divided into three fascial compartments: anterior, posterior and medial. The anterior compartment group of muscles mostly act to extend the knee, and include iliopsoas, quadriceps femoris (vastus lateralis/intermedius/medialis, rectus femoris), sartorius and pectineus. These muscles are innervated by the femoral nerve (L2–L4). The medial compartment group of muscles are the hip adductors, and include gracilis, obturator externus, adductor brevis, adductor longus and adductor magnus. These muscles are innervated by the obturator nerve, a branch from the lumbar plexus. The posterior compartment group of muscles are the hamstrings, and include the biceps femoris, semitendinosus and semimembranosus. These muscles are innervated by the sciatic nerve (L4–S3) and extend the hip and flex the knee. Subcutaneous and intramuscular injection of drugs is a major risk factor for abscess formation, as in this patient's case.

☑ 3a Ciprofloxacin 400 mg BD + Clindamycin 600 mg QDS + Benzylpenicillin 1.2 g QDS

Prior to identification and sensitivities, this patient needs to be covered with broad-spectrum antibiotics with both Gram-positive and Gram-negative cover. Ciprofloxacin is a quinolone that has predominant Gram-negative cover, particularly for *Haemophilus* and

Neisseria species. Clindamycin is a macrolide that is active against Gram-positive cocci, including *streptococci* and penicillin-resistant staphylococci, and many anaerobes, especially *Bacteroides fragilis*. Benzylpenicillin is a penicillin with good efficacy against many streptococcal, gonococcal and meningococcal infections. This combination provides the broadest cover for multiple Gram-positive and Gram-negative organisms and is most appropriate as initial cover. Rationalisation should then be done once the organisms are fully identified and sensitivities known alongside advice from local Microbiologists. Flucloxacillin is used for infections caused by penicillin-resistant staphylococci and is generally used for simple skin infections like cellulitis, erysipelas, secondary bacterial infection of eczema and infective endocarditis combined with additional antimicrobials. Metronidazole is highly active against certain Gram-negative and anaerobic species.

KEY LEARNING POINTS

- Be cautious of deep infections in high-risk patients such as intravenous drug users. Imaging modalities such as ultrasound and MRI can help delineate the extent of infection in conjunction with biochemical markers.
- Specific MRI protocols such as proton-weighted sequences can help non-invasively delineate if there is any joint involvement and help with surgical planning.
- Broad-antimicrobial cover is essential in treating these infections. Local guidelines should be followed.

Thunderclap headache

A 60-year-old man presents to the emergency department with a sudden onset severe headache that began immediately after intercourse the previous night. The pain was initially frontal, radiating posteriorly with neck stiffness, and reported as 10/10 severity 'like being hit in the head by a brick'. There was associated nausea but no vomiting. The pain is worse on coughing. He denies any facial droop, problems with speech or limb weakness. He denies use of phosphodiesterase inhibitors. Past medical history includes hypertension and gastro-oesophageal reflux disease.

Initial observations are recorded as HR 99, BP 188/91, SpO$_2$ 98% on room air, RR 17, temperature 36.7°C (98.1°F), GCS 15/15. Although the patient is clearly in pain, your examination is otherwise normal with no findings on full neurological examination.

A non-contrast CT head is performed.

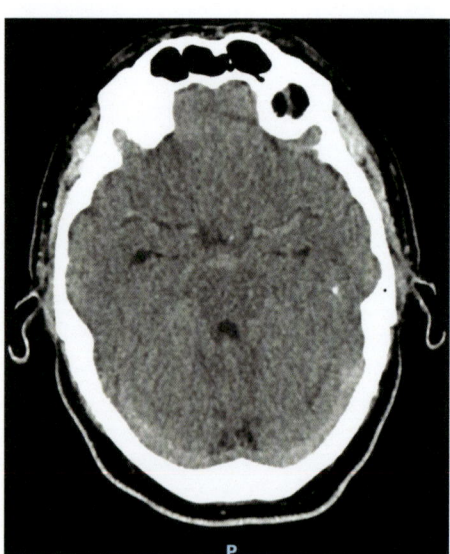

DOI: 10.1201/9781003461456-66

1. Which of the following is NOT a risk factor for the displayed diagnosis?

   a. Hypertension

   b. Autosomal dominant polycystic kidney disease (ADPKD)

   c. Female sex

   d. Connective tissue disorders, (for example, Marfan's disease)

   e. High-dose steroids

2. Which of the following is the most common site for aneurysms that may lead to the above?

   a. Anterior communicating artery (ACOM)

   b. Posterior communicating artery (PCOM)

   c. Middle cerebral artery (MCA)

   d. Basilar artery

   e. Internal carotid artery

3. Which one of the following medications is used to prevent secondary ischaemic injury in the above?

   a. Sodium nitroprusside infusion 0.5–1.5 mcg/kg/minute IV

   b. Magnesium sulphate 4 g IV over 20 minutes

   c. Nimodipine 60 mg PO or NG

   d. Labetalol 50 mg IV bolus

   e. Diclofenac 100 mg PR

☑ 1e High-dose steroids

The CT shows fresh blood in the interpeduncular and prepontine cisterns and in the superior cervical spinal canal; these appearances are consistent with acute subarachnoid haemorrhage (SAH). Non-contrast CT has a sensitivity of 98% within 12 hours. Risk factors for SAH include female sex (especially post-menopausal), age >50 years, smoking, use of the combined oral contraceptive pill, alcohol abuse, hypertension, connective tissue disorders, ADPKD, personal or family history of aneurysms and coarctation of the aorta (which commonly occurs in connective tissue disorders such as Marfan's). 'Coital cephalgia' or primary headache associated with sexual activity (PHASA), which is a headache associated with sexual intercourse, could be a differential diagnosis with this presentation. It has a prevalence of around 1–1.5% and is more common in males and individuals with migraine, tension-type headache and benign exertional headache. However, this is a diagnosis of exclusion and you must investigate the patient for SAH if there is clinical suspicion including lumbar puncture to examine for CSF xanthochromia if the initial CT does not demonstrate bleeding.

☑ 2b Posterior communicating artery (PCOM)

SAH can be aneurysmal (85%) or non-aneurysmal. If aneurysmal, it is typically due to a rupture of the saccular or berry aneurysm or rarely a mycotic aneurysm. Aneurysmal disease is associated with ADPKD, connective tissue disorders, atherosclerosis and hypertension. The sites of aneurysms are most commonly in PCOM (40%), followed by ACOM (35%), MCA (20%), vertebrobasilar (4%) and, rarely, the internal carotid artery. Non-aneurysmal SAH may be due to trauma, arteriovenous malformation, neoplasm, angioma or cortical thrombosis. Given the evidence of acute bleeding on the non-contrast CT head, further imaging with CT angiography should be performed, which could identify the bleeding point or the presence and location of an aneurysm.

☑ 3c Nimodipine 60 mg PO or NG

Initial management of SAH aims to treat and prevent further bleeding and to reduce the rate of secondary complications, such as cerebral ischaemia or hydrocephalus. Re-bleeding is the most imminent danger; a first aim in ruptured aneurysmal SAH is therefore occlusion of the aneurysm. 'Coiling', i.e. endovascular obliteration by means of platinum spirals, is now the preferred mode of treatment, but some patients require a direct neurosurgical approach and 'clipping' when coiling is not suitable, for example, wide necked aneurysm, presence of blood clot or rupture of a previously coiled aneurysm. Other ways to reduce risk of re-bleeding is avoidance of hypertension, no coughing or Valsalva, and sedation if required. Another complication is delayed cerebral ischaemia due to vasospasm; the risk is reduced with oral nimodipine (60 mg PO 4-hourly) and by maintaining circulatory volume. Secondary hydrocephalus might cause gradual obtundation in the first few hours or days and can be treated by lumbar puncture or external ventricular drainage (EVD) depending on the site of obstruction. Do also remember that you may note abnormalities on other routine investigations. The ECG may demonstrate repolarisation abnormalities in the heart leading to peaked T waves, ST depression and QT prolongation; hyponatraemia may indicate SIADH or cerebral salt wasting, which worsens vasospasm; and chest radiograph can demonstrate neurogenic pulmonary oedema.

KEY LEARNING POINTS

- Multi-axial CT scanning is 98% sensitive for subarachnoid haemorrhage if performed within 12 hours of headache onset.
- Primary headache associated with sexual activity (PHASA) is a diagnosis of exclusion and you must investigate to rule out SAH first.
- Proceed to a CT angiogram, preferably at the same time as the primary CT head scan if subarachnoid haemorrhage is detected, in order to look for aneurysms and active bleeding sites.

Transient loss of consciousness

A 21-year-old man is brought in by his father, having had multiple 'collapses'. The patient informs you he drank around 10 pints of beer at a pub with friends before cycling home and recalls falling off his bike on the way. He cannot remember the fall but knows his father picked him up and took him home. He collapsed at home whilst attempting to go to the toilet and had one further collapse on arrival of the ambulance crew.

A primary survey is performed:

1. Airway: maintaining own airway, no cervical spine pain noted
2. Breathing: RR 22, SpO$_2$ 100% on room air, normal work of breathing, no chest wall deformity/bruising/tenderness, equal air entry bilaterally
3. Circulation: HR 65, BP 121/58, peripheral capillary refill time 3 seconds, no evidence of external haemorrhage
4. Disability: GCS 15/15, PEARLA 3 mm/3 mm
5. Exposure: there is abdominal tenderness with guarding in the left upper quadrant, pelvis stable, no long bone deformity, temperature 35°C (95°F)

1. According to the Advanced Trauma Life Support (ATLS) classification, what class of hypovolaemic shock would this patient fit?
   a. Class I
   b. Class II
   c. Class III
   d. Class IV
   e. Class V

DOI: 10.1201/9781003461456-67

A trauma series CT is performed with the abdominal series shown.

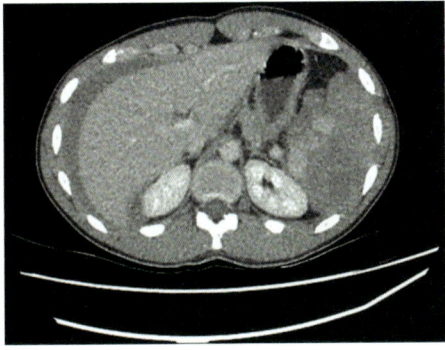

2. What is the best description of the findings this CT scan shows?

    a. Grade IV spleen injury (50% devascularisation) with free fluid/bleeding in the abdomen

    b. Grade IV spleen injury (75% devascularisation) with free fluid/bleeding into the abdomen

    c. Grade III spleen injury (intraparenchymal or subcapsular haematoma) with free fluid in the abdomen

    d. Grade V spleen injury (shattered spleen) and Grade III liver laceration

    e. Grade V spleen injury (shattered spleen) with gross haematoperitoneum

Following the scan, the patient is moved to the resuscitation room.

After warming with a forced air warming blanket, you note his BP has dropped slightly to 100/50 mmHg and HR is now 111 bpm.

3. What is the best set of steps to optimally manage this patient?

    a. Give 1 g tranexamic acid (TXA) IV, catheterise, transfer to intensive care unit (ICU) for invasive blood pressure monitoring and conservative management

    b. Give 1 g TXA IV, resuscitate with warmed balanced crystalloid, prepare for transfer to the off-site interventional radiology suite

    c. Give 1 g TXA IV, catheterise, activate major haemorrhage protocol, ring the senior general surgeon for urgent laparotomy

    d. Give 1 g TXA IV, catheterise, resuscitate with warmed balanced crystalloid, turn off the forced air warmer, monitor in the resuscitation room

    e. Give 1 g TXA IV, catheterise, resuscitate with colloid to stabilise BP, ring the senior general surgeon for laparotomy

☑ **1a Class I**

Recognising shock can be one of the most difficult aspects in the management of an injured patient. In the early assessment period, shock is identified by signs of end-organ hypoperfusion on examination and with point-of-care measures. The ATLS classification of hypovolaemic shock is based on vital signs of heart rate (HR), blood pressure (BP), pulse pressure (PP), respiratory rate (RR), urine output (UO), GCS, and base deficit (BE, mEq/L), and estimated blood loss (EBL) in percentage terms. A total circulating volume accounts is approximately 7% of body weight, so according to ATLS, the following is for a 70 kg person:

- Class I: EBL up to 750 mL or <15%. Generally, the clinical observations are within normal limits and the BE is within normal range (+2 to –2). This is true of our patient scenario above.
- Class II: EBL 750 to 1500 mL or 15–30%. HR 100–120, PP narrows slightly with normal to slightly decreased systolic BP, RR normal, GCS normally unimpaired but may be mildly anxious, BE –2 to –6.
- Class III: EBL 1500 to 2000 mL or 30–40%. HR 120–140, RR 20–30, systolic BP decreased with narrowed PP, UO decreased 5–15 mL/hour, may be anxious or confused, BE –6 to –10.
- Class IV: EBL >2000 mL or >40%. HR >140, RR >35, systolic BP decreased with narrowed PP, UO <5 mL/hour, confused and lethargic, BE –10 or less.
- 'Class V': does not exist in the ATLS classification.

☑ **2e Grade V spleen injury (shattered spleen) with gross haematoperitoneum**

The CT shows a shattered spleen with free fluid in the abdomen, highly suggestive of active bleeding, which constitutes an American Association for the Surgery of Trauma (AAST) Grade V splenic injury. Grades I–III splenic injuries are based on the size of any visualised parenchymal lacerations and subcapsular and/or intraparenchymal haematoma; these are generally managed non-operatively. If there is evidence of splenic vascular injury or active bleeding into the peritoneum, this automatically means the injury seen is at least a Grade IV. A Grade V injury is a shattered spleen with vascular injury. Non-operative management may be trialled in patients with haemodynamic stability and isolated splenic injuries irrespective of injury grade following blunt trauma in some centres if they have capability for intensive monitoring and angiography and embolisation. However, Grade IV and V injuries are more typically associated with haemodynamic instability and or additional intra-abdominal injuries, which should prompt operative management.

☑ 3c Give 1 g TXA IV, catheterise, activate major haemorrhage protocol, ring the senior general surgeon for urgent laparotomy

This patient is now cardiovascularly unstable: BP has dropped and the HR risen. In this context, this must be assumed to be due to decompensated hypovolaemic shock and not from warming the patient. TXA is advised in major trauma since the CRASH-2 trial in 2010; although a small absolute risk reduction in mortality was shown with TXA it was associated with minimal adverse effects. The definitive management in this patient's injury with associated haemodynamic instability is surgical management with laparotomy and splenectomy. He may require rapid blood replacement, either in the resuscitation room if he decompensates or in theatre, and so the major haemorrhage protocol should be activated. There is a careful balance of trying to raise the blood pressure too quickly, which may paradoxically make bleeding worse, and maintaining organ perfusion. Angiography and embolisation may be offered to suitable patients with vascular abnormalities or higher-grade injuries, and the aim is reduction in rates of laparotomy and splenectomy. Though it can be successful, the bleeding point is not always identified and even if embolisation is performed, some patients still require surgery.

KEY LEARNING POINTS

- ATLS gives a structured approach to classifying haemorrhagic shock based on physiological and biochemical parameters. Blood pressure does not drop until significant volume loss in most patients.
- Splenic injuries are graded by the American Association for the Surgery of Trauma (AAST) ranging from Grade I (minimal bleeding) to Grade V (shattered spleen).
- Do not ignore worsening of physiological parameters in the trauma patients. As part of the treatment, definitive haemorrhage control should be sought as well as restoration of blood volume.

CASE 68

Trauma to the chest

A 23-year-old male is dropped off at the emergency department (ED). You are working in a hospital that is not a major trauma centre. He states he has been out celebrating during lockdown and has been drinking alcohol and has taken some 'balloons'. Approximately 15 minutes ago, he was stabbed to the left chest underneath the nipple. He alleges not to have seen the assailant or the size of the blade and has been walked into the resuscitation room. He looks pale and diaphoretic. There is approximately 100 mL of blood on his chest and trousers and the wound is being compressed by the patient. A trauma team is present.

Initial observations are recorded as HR 110, BP 134/60, SpO$_2$ 98% on room air, RR 31, GCS 15/15.

1. Which of the following best describes how you are going to proceed?
   a. Undress the patient, perform a 360-degree stab check, transfer the patient to the trolley, perform a primary survey, insert a line and draw bloods, perform an eFAST scan and focused echo
   b. Ask the patient to lie on the trolley, apply 3-point immobilisation of the cervical spine, perform a primary survey, insert a line and draw bloods, order a lateral neck radiograph
   c. Ask the patient to lie on the trolley, apply a semi-rigid collar, perform a primary survey, insert a line and draw bloods, order a CT chest with contrast
   d. Ask the patient to lie on the trolley, apply 3-point immobilisation of the cervical spine, perform a primary survey, insert a line and draw bloods, order a supine chest radiograph
   e. Undress the patient, ask the patient to lie on the trolley, administer 4 mg IV lorazepam when he refuses to do so in 'best interests'

Inspection of the chest reveals a single 4 cm wound under the left nipple.

A venous blood gas (VBG) has been processed and reveals pH 7.173, pCO$_2$ 4.7, HCO$_3^-$ 13.4, BE −15.3, Hb 14.8, Lactate 15, Glucose 8.

DOI: 10.1201/9781003461456-68

A point-of-care focused echocardiogram is performed as part of his assessment.

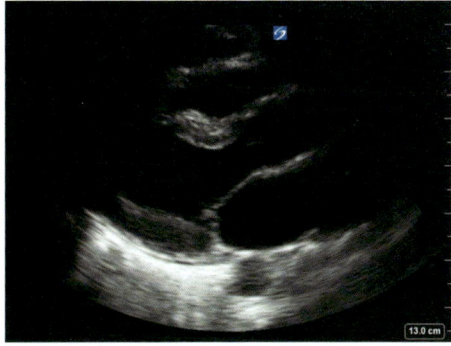

2. Which of the following is the best description of what this shows?

   a. Normal

   b. Mitral valve leaflet disruption

   c. Right ventricle laceration

   d. Descending thoracic aorta injury

   e. Haemopericardium

3. Which of the following is the best description of how you would proceed with this patient's management based on your findings so far?

   a. 1 g tranexamic acid IV, admit under general surgeons locally

   b. 1 g tranexamic acid IV, CT polytrauma scan, refer to cardiology

   c. Instil local anaesthetic, probe and explore the wound and close, admit for observation under general surgeons locally

   d. 1 g tranexamic acid IV, perform a time-critical transfer to the regional major trauma centre for further management

   e. 1 g tranexamic acid IV, CT polytrauma scan, call regional major trauma centre to review imaging and await response

☑ 1a Undress the patient, perform a 360-degree stab check, transfer the patient to the trolley, perform a primary survey, insert a line and draw bloods, perform an eFAST scan and focused echo

This patient has a very specific injury and needs a modification of the standard Advanced Trauma Life Support (ATLS) protocol. These patients commonly walk into the ED after being dropped off outside. This is the best time to perform a 'stab check'; rapidly and sensitively undress the patient and perform a 360-degree check of the patient to exclude any additional wounds. Gang culture will often deliberately target the buttocks (as a form of humiliation, but this risks damage to iliac vessels), chest and axillae. After performing the stab check, allow the patient to lie on the bed semi-recumbent and perform a rapid primary survey with an ABCDE assessment. During the primary survey ensure to obtain 2 x IV cannula and draw bloods including VBG, FBC, U&Es, coagulation screen and group & screen. As the location of this injury is very high risk for myocardial damage, you may proceed to a rapid point-of-care eFAST scan and a focused echo. This will allow you to assess for evidence of intra-abdominal or pericardial fluid. Often this can be achieved faster than a portable chest radiograph but should there be signs of a pneumothorax clinically do not delay the portable chest radiograph to assess size. If clinical features of tension pneumothorax are present, immediate decompression is indicated and you should not wait for a chest radiograph. Note that this patient did have a 2 mm pneumothorax.

☑ 2e Haemopericardium

This is a parasternal long axis view (PLAX) of the heart. The large cavity in the centre of the image is the left ventricle with the mitral valve above it opening and closing. The mechanism of injury is highly suggestive of ventricular injury as the left nipple corresponds to the anatomical landmark for the apex of the heart. If you look very carefully, there is a flash of free fluid just above the bright line of the pericardium, which in this context must be assumed to be haemopericardium. This patient was scanned rapidly, and other views confirmed the presence and persistence of this fluid. Remember that this patient presented only 15 minutes post-injury and so significant fluid may not have accumulated yet. The descending aorta is the round structure at the bottom middle of the image and is normal. And the mitral valve is functioning normally. Again, all of these structures can be potentially injured with this type of injury.

☑ 3d 1 g tranexamic acid IV, perform a time-critical transfer to the regional major trauma centre for further management

Based on the finding that there is an early pericardial effusion, the best management would be to transfer this patient to the regional major trauma centre (MTC) without further delay. Often these patients slowly continue to leak blood. Therefore, delays at the local site waiting for CT scans to be performed and then contacting the MTC for an opinion puts the patient at risk of sudden death from a cardiac tamponade. In addition, young patients will compensate physiologically until the last minute and then suddenly suffer cardiac arrest. Should this occur then activate a major haemorrhage and adult cardiac arrest call, rapidly fill the patient and proceed to a clamshell thoracotomy immediately instead of CPR. The aim of the clamshell thoracotomy is to decompress the chest for potential tension pneumothorax, halve the circulation by manual compression of the aorta (performed once the chest is opened), relieve the heart of pericardial tamponade by opening the pericardium and to repair any bleeding vessels (intercostal vessels, left internal mammary artery) or repair ventricular lacerations by direct occlusion, insertion of a Foley urinary catheter or direct suture.

KEY LEARNING POINTS

- Stab wounds should be taken seriously; entry wounds should be regarded carefully as the size of laceration may not correspond to depth of wound or structures injured.
- Point-of-care ultrasound can be a very useful adjunct, especially when cardiac injury is suspected.
- Do not delay the transfer of critically unwell patients with haemopericardium, as clinical course can be unpredictable and these patients may suddenly decompensate in the ED.

Vomiting and ECG changes

A 28-year-old woman presents to the emergency department (ED) with recurrent vomiting for 4 days. She feels very thirsty, has tingling around her face and mouth, complains of leg cramps and is finding it increasingly difficult to walk. She states that she is under investigation for a 'condition' but investigations were paused due to the COVID-19 pandemic.

Initial observations are recorded as HR 72, BP 107/73, SpO$_2$ 100% on room air, RR 18, temperature 36.5°C (97.7°F), GCS 15/15, capillary blood glucose 5.8 mmol/L. You note that the patient looks dehydrated and that her skin turgor is reduced. Cardiovascular, respiratory, abdominal and neurological examinations are normal.

You review the ECG.

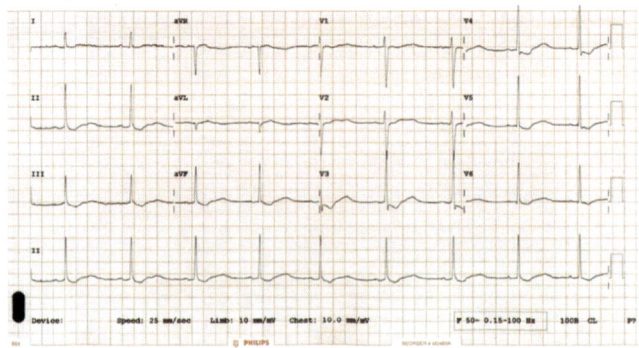

1. What abnormalities are shown and what electrolyte disturbance does this suggest?
   a. Prolonged QU interval, flattened T waves, U waves – hypokalaemia
   b. Prolonged QTc, tall-tented T waves – hyperkalaemia
   c. Prolonged QTc, normal T waves – hypocalcaemia
   d. Prolonged QTc, flattened T waves, U waves – hypermagnesaemia
   e. Prolonged QTc, normal T waves – hypercalcaemia

The patient continues to feel nauseous.

Initial bloods have been taken and are in progress. Point-of-care venous blood gas is being re-run and there is a delay due to recalibration of the machine.

DOI: 10.1201/9781003461456-69

Urinary β-hCG test is outstanding.

2. Which antiemetic would you NOT prescribe given the above ECG?
    a. Cyclizine 50 mg IV
    b. Prochlorperazine 12.5 mg IM
    c. Ondansetron 4 mg IV
    d. Metoclopramide 10 mg IV
    e. Nabilone 1 mg PO

3. Which disorder would NOT account for this electrolyte imbalance?
    a. Gietelman syndrome
    b. Conn's syndrome
    c. Bartter's syndrome
    d. Addison's disease
    e. Cushing's syndrome

☑ 1a Prolonged QU interval, flattened T waves, U waves – hypokalaemia

This ECG shows the following changes: an apparent prolonged QTc interval at 529 ms (upper range 440 in men, 450 in women), flat T waves and the presence of U waves. The apparent prolonged QTc interval is actually a QU interval due to fusion of U and T waves. This is classical for severe hypokalaemia and this patient's potassium was 1.7 mmol/L on formal laboratory blood test. If these ECG changes are seen, move the patient to the resuscitation room ideally or a visible monitored environment, place on a cardiac monitor, and replace both potassium and magnesium, along with any other electrolytes. Typical changes in other electrolyte abnormalities are: (1) Hyperkalaemia – prolonged PR interval, flat P waves, tall-tented T waves, widening QRS complexes, VF/VT, AV block, the 'sine wave of death', asystole; (2) Hypocalcaemia – prolonged QTC but normal T waves; (3) Hypercalcaemia – shortened QTc, J (Osborn) waves; (4) Hypermagnesaemia – as per hyperkalaemia.

☑ 2c Ondansetron 4 mg IV

From the list of options presented, ondansetron should be used with caution in patients with hypokalaemia. There is case-reported evidence of ondansetron causing severe hypokalaemia. The mechanism seems to lie within the nephron whereby inhibits the Na^+-K^+-2Cl^- transporter at the loop of Henle and then upregulates the Na^+-K^+-ATPase throughout the nephron. The other major group of patients in which ondansetron should be avoided is patients with a true prolonged QTc due to the risk of further elongation and potential deterioration totorsades de pointes. Risk is dose related and highest when using the injectable form of ondansetron. High-risk groups of patients presenting to the ED include those at high risk of electrolyte disturbance (alcohol excess, vomiting, gastroenteritis, metabolic disorders), cardiac patients and congenital disorders such as congenital long QT syndrome. Take care to scrutinise electrolytes rapidly available on the venous blood gas (VBG) and ECG before prescribing antiemetics. For the other antiemetics listed, watch out for acute dystonic reaction with metoclopramide (particularly in young women and the elderly), tachycardia and thrombophlebitis with cyclizine, drowsiness with prochlorperazine and hallucinations or euphoria with nabilone; this is a cannabinoid used for nausea and vomiting in chemotherapy patients.

☑ 3d Addison's disease

Possible causes of hypokalaemia include: Gitelman syndrome, Bartter's syndrome, Conn's syndrome and Cushing's syndrome. Addison's disease typically causes low sodium and high potassium levels and is associated with clinical features of low blood pressure and prominent palmar creases or darkened skin tone. Gitelman syndrome and Bartter's syndrome are rare hereditary hypokalaemic tubulopathies. Gietelman syndrome is an autosomal recessive disorder with a specific set of channel mutations affecting the renal tubule causing loss of sodium, magnesium, chloride and potassium. Characteristically these patients can present with hypochloraemic metabolic alkalosis and hypokalaemia. Heterozygote carriers are often asymptomatic, but some report muscle cramps and weakness. Bartter's syndrome is a disorder where a mutation affects potassium transport at the thick ascending loop of Henle. Patients present with hypokalaemia and hypercalciuria with some patients at increased risk of renal stones. Conn's syndrome (primary hyperaldosteronism) classically causes hypokalaemia and hypertension. Look for high aldosterone levels and normal to low plasma renin activity – this can be assessed with the aldosterone to renin ratio measurement. Cushing's syndrome can cause hypokalaemia due to ectopic adrenocorticotropic hormone (ACTH) secretion, which results in high aldosterone levels. Along with hypokalaemia, look for hypernatraemia and hypertension.

KEY LEARNING POINTS

- Characteristic ECG changes of moderate to severe hypokalaemia include a prolongation of the PR-interval, an apparent prolonged QT interval, flattened T waves and U waves.
- Certain medications can worsen hypokalaemia, such as ondansetron, or interact with cardiac conduction, particularly in states of prolonged QTc.
- Addison's disease characteristically causes hyperkalaemia in conjunction with hypoglycaemia and hyponatraemia.

Wound problem

A 62-year-old woman attends the emergency department with her daughter. You have been asked to see her after she was initially directed to the urgent treatment centre. She complains of a 10-day history of painful discharging wounds on her left foot. On further questioning, you find she has had non-painful wounds present on the foot for months, for which she has been self-managing with dressings. She now walks with a limp, but otherwise is systemically well. She has recently arrived in the UK from Senegal. Past medical history includes hypertension and type 2 diabetes mellitus.

Initial observations are recorded as HR 79, BP 133/63, SpO$_2$ 99% on room air, RR 18, temperature 37.0°C (98.6°F), CBG 5.5.

A photo of the wound is shown.

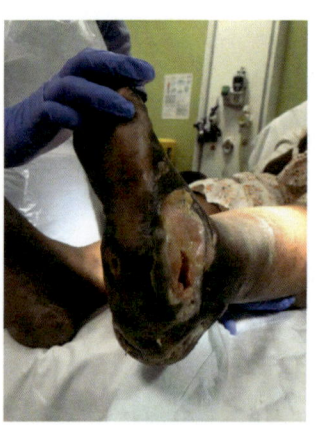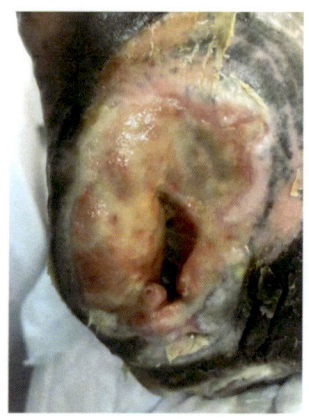

1. What is the single most likely underlying cause of this presentation?
   a. Poorly controlled diabetes
   b. Chronic venous insufficiency
   c. Pyoderma gangrenosum
   d. *Mycobacterium leprae*
   e. Marjolin's ulcer

DOI: 10.1201/9781003461456-70

Radiographs of the foot and ankle are requested.

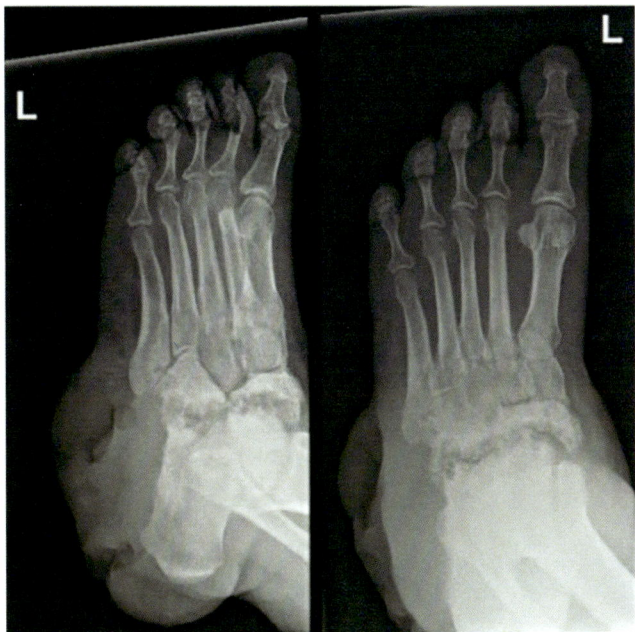

2. What is the likely cause of this appearance?

   a. Osteomyelitis of the midfoot

   b. Chondrosarcoma

   c. Charcot arthropathy

   d. Paget's disease of the bone

   e. Fracture of the navicular and cuboid

3. Which of the following describes the most common type of the above abnormality according to Brodsky classification?

   a. Type 1

   b. Type 2

   c. Type 3

   d. Type 4

   e. Type 5

☑ 1a Poorly controlled diabetes

The history of a long-standing painless wound suggests an element of neuropathic ulceration, which is commonly associated with poorly controlled diabetes mellitus. If the wound has since become painful, with increased discharge, this could be suggestive of superimposed infection or other complication related to the neuropathic ulcer. Neuropathic ulcers are mostly located over pressure points, such as heels, toes or base of great toe. In response to pressure, skin increases in thickness, but minor injury causes this to break down and ulcerate. The list of differential diagnoses for skin wounds/ulcers is wide, but some clinical characteristics can point you towards the correct diagnosis. Leg ulceration most commonly occurs after a minor injury in association with venous insufficiency (45–80%), chronic arterial insufficiency (5–20%), diabetes mellitus (15–25%) and hypertension. Other chronic ulcers may be skin cancer, a symptom of systemic disease such as systemic sclerosis, vasculitis or pyoderma gangrenosum and infection. With the history of living abroad, remember to consider tropical causes such as leprosy and cutaneous tuberculosis.

☑ 2c Charcot arthropathy

Charcot's foot is the alternative term for 'diabetic foot'. It is a consequence of neuropathy and impaired circulation often seen with diabetes. The bones become weakened and as a result traumatic injuries are more common with minimal force, plus neuropathy means this trauma may not be perceived by the patient. Continuing to walk on the affected foot can lead to further fractures, non-union or mal-union and joint dislocations. The combination of bone disintegration and trauma can warp and deform the shape of the foot, leading to Charcot arthropathy. Early osteomyelitis may only show soft tissue swelling; after 10–14 days in adults, you may see regional osteopenia, periosteal reactions/thickening, loss of trabecular bone architecture and new bone apposition. Paget's disease is a disease of bone remodelling leading to abnormally shaped, weak and brittle bones. It most commonly affects the axial skeleton. Chondrosarcoma is a malignancy of cartilage matrix-forming cells, most commonly affecting the pelvis, ribs, humerus, scapula, proximal femur and tibia. It most commonly affects individuals over 40 years old, and slightly more often in men. Radiographic features are lytic lesions with intralesional calcifications, and endosteal scalloping.

☑ 3a Type 1

The Brodsky classification is based on the joints affected by Charcot arthropathy and is split into 5 types, with type 1 being most common (~60%). Type 1 involves tarsometatarsal and naviculocuneiform joints, leading to rocker-bottom feet with valgus angulation. Type 2 involves subtalar, talonavicular or calcaneocuboid joints. Type 3A involves the tibiotalar joint and type 3B follows fracture of calcaneal tuberosity. Type 4 involves a combination of areas and type 5 occurs in the forefoot only. Complex diabetic feet need careful management from a multidisciplinary team, including multiple special- ties. infectious diseases, orthopaedics and vascular Surgery will need to be involved with this patient. Infectious diseases, alongside microbiology, will be able to advise regarding treating tissue infection and osteomyelitis as well as providing advice about tropical infections such as leprosy. Orthopaedics (joint) and vascular surgeons (duplex assessment) will both need to assess the foot to determine any surgical intervention, for example debridement or amputation. With the severity of disease in this patient, she may end up requiring amputation. Other members of the multidisciplinary team will be tissue viability nurses (wound care, vacuum-assisted closure dressings) and podiatry.

KEY LEARNING POINTS

- Poorly controlled diabetes can result in peripheral neuropathy resulting in chronic ulceration and destruction of the joint – Charcot arthropathy.
- Classical radiograph changes of Charcot arthropathy encompass three phases known as the Eichenholtz classification: 1. fragmentation and dissolution; 2. co-alescence and fusion of fragments; 3. reconstitution.
- The Brodsky classification is used to classify Charcot neuroarthropathy.

APPENDIX 1
Vital signs normal values

Vital signs		Normal range & units
HR	Heart rate	60 – 100 beats per minute
BP	Blood pressure	90/60 – 120/80 mmHg
SpO$_2$	Oxygen saturation	94 – 98% (on room air)
RR	Respiratory rate	12 – 20 breaths per minute
Temp	Temperature	36.1 – 37.2 °C (97 – 99 F)
GCS	Glasgow Coma Scale	
	Eye opening response	4 Spontaneously open
		3 To sound
		2 To pressure
		1 No response
	Verbal response	5 Orientated to time, place and person
		4 Confused
		3 Words
		2 Sounds
		1 No response
	Motor response	6 Obeys commands
		5 Localising
		4 Normal flexion
		3 Abnormal flexion
		2 Extension
		1 No response

Paediatrics

	HR	RR	Systolic BP
3 months	110 – 180	30 – 45	70 - 105
6 months	110 – 180	25 – 35	72 – 110
1 to 3 years	80 – 140	20 – 30	74 – 110
3 to 5 years	80 – 120	20 – 26	78 – 112
5 to 8 years	75 – 110	18 – 22	82 – 115

APPENDIX 2
Laboratory test normal values

Laboratory test		Normal range & units (UK)	Normal range & units (US)
Hb	Haemoglobin	130–170 g/L	13–17 g/dL
WCC	White cell count	3.0–10.0 × 10⁹/L	4000– 1000/µL
MCV	Mean corpuscular volume	80–99 fL	80–100 µm³
Plt	Platelet count	150–400 × 10⁹/L	150–400 × 10³/µL
Neuts	Neutrophil count	2.0–7.5 × 10⁹/L	2000–8250/µL
Na⁺	Sodium	135–145 mmol/L	13 –145 mEq/L
K⁺	Potassium	3.5–5.1 mmol/L	3.5–5.1 mEq/L
Urea	Urea	1.7–8.3 mmol/L	8–25 mg/dL
Cr	Creatinine	66–112 mmol/L	0.5–1.1 mg/dL
eGFR	Estimate glomerular filtration rate	>60 mLl/min/1.73 m²	
CRP	C-reactive protein	0–50 g/L	0.8–1.0 mg/dL
Bili	Bilirubin	0–20 µmol/L	0.0–1.0 mg/dL
AST	Aspartate aminotransferase	10–40 IU/L	
ALT	Alanine transaminase	10–50 IU/L	
ALP	Alkaline phosphatase	40–129 IU/L	
Alb	Albumin	34–50 g/L	3.0–5.0 g/dL
Amylase	Amylase	40–140 U/L	
Ca²⁺	Calcium	2.1–2.6 mmol/L	8.5–10.5 mg/dL
PO₄³⁻	Phosphate	0.80–1.50 mmol/L	2.5–4.5 mg/dL
INR	International normalised ratio	0.8–1.1	
Troponin T	Troponin T	<14 ng/L	<15 ng/mL
D-dimer	D-dimer	<500 ng/mL	<0.5 µg/mL
TSH	Thyroid stimulating hormone	0.2–4.0 mIU/L	
T4	Levothyroxine	10–20 pmol/L	5.0–12.0 µg/dL
CBG	Capillary blood glucose	4.0–8.0 mmol/L	70–110 mg/dL

Laboratory test		Normal range & units (UK & US)	
		Arterial	Venous
pH	pH	7.35–7.45	7.3–7.41
pCO_2	Partial pressure carbon dioxide	4.7–6.0 kPa	5.5–6.8 kPa
		38–42 mmHg	42–53 mmHg
pO_2	Partial pressure oxygen	10.6–13.3 kPa	4.0–5.3 kPa
		75–100 mmHg	35–42 mmHg
HCO_3^-	Standard bicarbonate	22–28 mEq/L	
BE	Base excess	–2 to +2	
Lactate	Lactate	0. –2.2 mmol/L	

APPENDIX 3
Abbreviations

ABCDE	Airway, breathing, circulation, disability, exposure assessment
ABG	Arterial blood gas
ACS	Acute coronary syndrome
ACTH	Adrenocorticotropic hormone
ACOM	Anterior communicating artery
ADPKD	Autosomal dominant polycystic kidney disease
AF	Atrial fibrillation
AFB	Acid-fast bacilli
AFP	Alpha fetoprotein
AKI	Acute kidney injury
ANA	Antinuclear antibody
ANCA	Anti-neutrophil cytoplasm antibodies
AS	Aortic stenosis
ATP	Adenosine triphosphate
AV	Atrioventricular node
AV	Aortic valve
AVM	Arteriovenous malformation
AVNRT	Atrioventricular nodal re-entrant tachycardia
AVRT	Atrioventricular re-entrant tachycardia
β-hCG	Beta-human chorionic gonadotropin
BD	Twice daily
BMI	Body mass index
BP	Blood pressure
bpm	Beats per minute
BPPV	Benign paroxysmal positional vertigo
Ca^{2+}	Calcium
CADASIL	Cerebral autosomal dominant arteriopathy
CBG	Capillary blood glucose
CHA_2DS_2-VASc	Atrial fibrillation stroke risk score
CJD	Creutzfeldt–Jakob disease
CMV	Cytomegalovirus
CNS	Central nervous system
COHb	Carboxyhaemoglobin
COPD	Chronic obstructive pulmonary disease
CPAP	Continuous positive airway pressure
CPP	Cryoprecipitate
CPR	Cardiopulmonary resuscitation
Cr	Creatinine
CRP	C-reactive protein
CRT	Capillary refill time
CSF	Cerebrospinal fluid
CT	Computerised tomography
CT KUB	CT kidneys, ureters & bladder
CTPA	CT pulmonary angiogram
CVC	Central venous catheter
DC	Direct current
DCM	Dilated cardiomyopathy
DIC	Disseminated intravascular coagulation
DOAC	Direct oral anticoagulant
DVT	Deep vein thrombosis
EBL	Estimated blood loss
EBV	Epstein–Barr virus
ECG	Electrocardiogram
ED	Emergency Department
EEG	Electroencephalogram
eGFR	Estimated glomerular filtration rate
eFAST	Extended focused assessment using sonography in trauma
EM	Erythema multiforme
ENA	Extractable nuclear antigen antibodies
ENT	Ear, nose and throat surgeons
ERCP	Endoscopic retrograde cholangiopancreatography
FBC	Full blood count
FFP	Fresh frozen plasma

FOOSH	Fall onto an outstretched hand	MC&S	Microscopy, culture & sensitivities
g	Gram	MCA	Middle cerebral artery
GABA	Gamma-aminobutyric acid	mcg	Microgram
GCS	Glasgow Coma Scale	mg	Milligram
GCTs	Germ cell tumours	Mg^{2+}	Magnesium
GI	Gastrointestinal	MI	Myocardial infarction
GP	General practitioner	mm	Millimetre
GTN	Glyceryl trinitrate	mph	Miles per hour
HASBLED	Score for major bleeding risk	MR	Mitral regurgitation
HASU	Hyperacute stroke unit	MRA	Magnetic resonance angiography
Hb	Haemoglobin	MRC	Medical Research Council
hCG	Human chorionic gonadotropin	MRCP	Magnetic resonance cholangiopancreatography
HE4	Human epididymis protein 4	MRI	Magnetic resonance imaging
HINTS	Head impulse, nystagmus, test of skew	MS	Multiple sclerosis
HIV	Human immunodeficiency virus	MSU	Midstream urine
HOCM	Hypertrophic obstructive cardiomyopathy	MTC	Major trauma centre
		Na^+	Sodium
HR	Heart rate	NAAT	Nucleic acid amplification test
HSV	Herpes simplex virus	NBM	Nil-by-mouth
HU	Hounsfield units	Neuts	Neutrophils
Hz	Hertz	NG	Nasogastric
ICP	Intracranial pressure	NMDA	N-methyl-D-aspartate
ICU	Intensive Care Unit	NOF	Neck of femur
IM	Intramuscular	NSAIDs	Non-steroidal anti-inflammatory drugs
INR	International normalised ratio		
IR	Interventional Radiology	O_2	Oxygen
ITP	Immune thrombocytopenia purpura	OD	Once daily
IV	Intravenous	OPG	Orthopantomogram
IVC	Inferior vena cava	ORIF	Open reduction and internal fixation
J	Joules	PA	Posterior-anterior
JVP	Jugular venous pressure	pCO_2	Partial pressure of carbon dioxide
K^+	Potassium	pO_2	Partial pressure of oxygen
kg	Kilogram	PCOM	Posterior communicating artery
LAD	Left anterior descending artery	PCR	Polymerase chain reaction
LAFB	Left anterior fascicular block	PE	Pulmonary embolism
LDH	Lactate dehydrogenase	PEA	Pulseless electrical activity
LFT	Liver function test	PEARLA	Pupils equal and reactive to light and accommodation
LMWH	Low molecular weight heparin		
LV	Left ventricle	PEEP	Positive end-expiratory pressure
LVH	Left ventricular hypertrophy	PET	Positron emission tomography
LVOT	Left ventricular outflow tract	PICA	Posterior inferior cerebellar artery
MAP	Mean arterial pressure	PLAX	Parasternal long axis
		PO	Oral

POCUS	Point-of-care ultrasound scan	sPESI	Simplified Pulmonary Embolism Severity Index
Ppeak	Peak airway pressure		
PRN	As required	SpO_2	Oxygen saturation
PSA	Prostate-specific antigen	SSP	Secondary spontaneous pneumothorax
PSAH	Pseudosubarachnoid haemorrhage		
PSAX	Parasternal short axis	STEMI	ST elevation myocardial infarction
PSP	Primary spontaneous pneumothorax	STP	Standard temperature and pressure
		SVT	Supraventricular tachycardia
PUD	Peptic ulcer disease	T2 FLAIR	T2-weighted Fluid Attenuated Inversion Recovery
PUJ	Pelvi-ureteric junction		
pVT	Pulseless ventricular tachycardia	TB	Tuberculosis
q-SOFA	Quick Sequential Organ Failure Assessment	TDS	Three times daily
		TEN	Toxic epidermal necrolysis
QDS	Four times daily	TIA	Transient ischaemic attack
RBBB	Right bundle branch block	TIPS	Transjugular intrahepatic portosystemic shunt
RCA	Right coronary artery		
RCC	Renal cell carcinoma	TLOC	Transient loss of consciousness
RR	Respiratory rate	TMJ	Temporomandibular joint
RRT	Renal replacement therapy	TR	Tricuspid regurgitation
RUSH-ED	Rapid ultrasound for shock & hypotension	TTE	Transthoracic echocardiogram
		TV	Tidal volume
RV	Right ventricle	TXA	Tranexamic acid
SAH	Subarachnoid haemorrhage	U&Es	Urea & electrolytes
SC	Subcutaneous	USS	Ultrasound scan
SHOCC	Sonography in hypotension & cardiac arrest	V/Q	Ventilation/perfusion
		VBG	Venous blood gas
SI	Sacroiliac	VF	Ventricular fibrillation
SIADH	Syndrome of inappropriate antidiuretic hormone	VT	Ventricular tachycardia
		VUJ	Vesicoureteric junction
SIMV	Synchronised-intermittent mechanical ventilation	VZV	Varicella zoster virus
		WCC	White cell count
SJS	Stevens–Johnson syndrome	WMH	White matter hyperintensity
SLE	Systemic lupus erythematous	XR	Radiograph

Index